Looking Through the Eyes of Nature

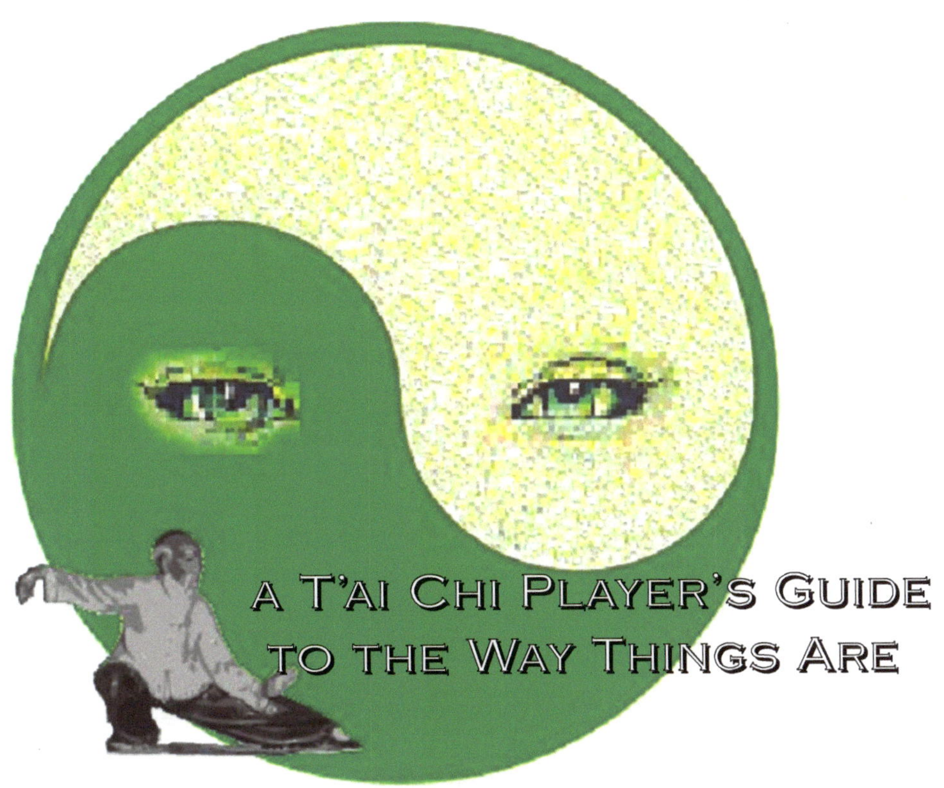

Max Wright

LOOKING THROUGH THE EYES OF NATURE

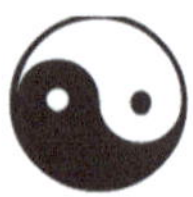

MAX WRIGHT

Published by 1stWorld Publishing
1100 North 4th St. Fairfield, Iowa 52556
tel: 641-209-5000 • fax: 641-209-3001
web: www.1stworldpublishing.com

First Edition

LCCN: 2007903157

SoftCover ISBN: 978-1-4218-9964-0

eBook ISBN: 978-1-4218-9966-4

Cover Design by Colin Davis

For my mother—who taught me all I know about my mother tongue—on the occasion of her 81st birthday.

Many thanks…

To my wife, Teresa Teravainen, and my dear friend, Colin Davis, for their support, encouragement and great work of arranging the text to make it more accessible. Without their help and vision this work would not have seen the light of day.

To friends and publishers Rodney and Nandini Charles for their inspiration to get the project under way in the first place.

And to my daughter, Robyn, and also to friends Jim Mileti, Bill Mandrell, Jeffrey and Linda Hedquist, and Bob Slifkin for their encouragement, technical suggestions, and patient proof reading.

CONTENTS

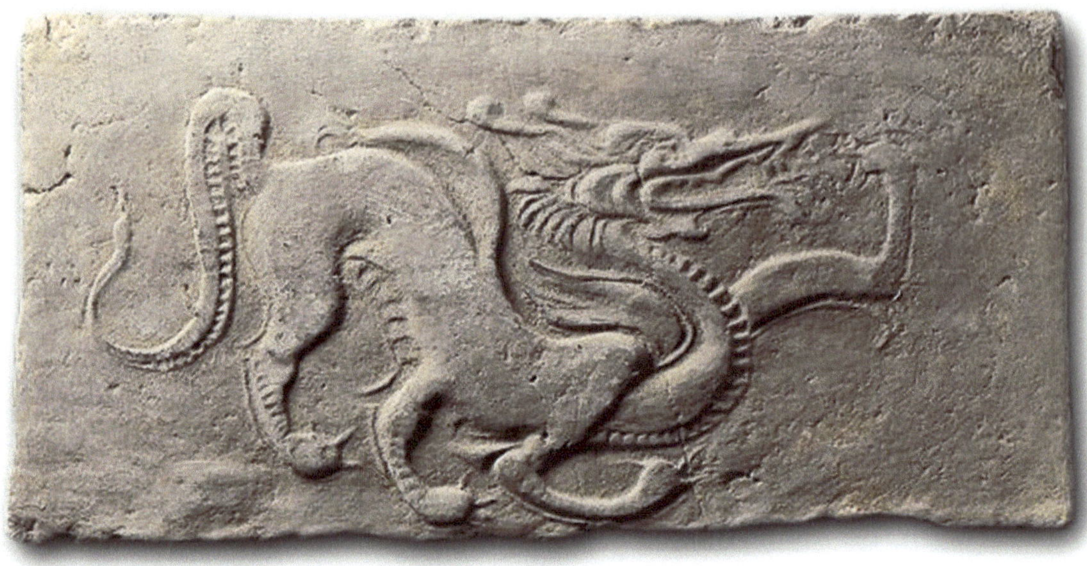

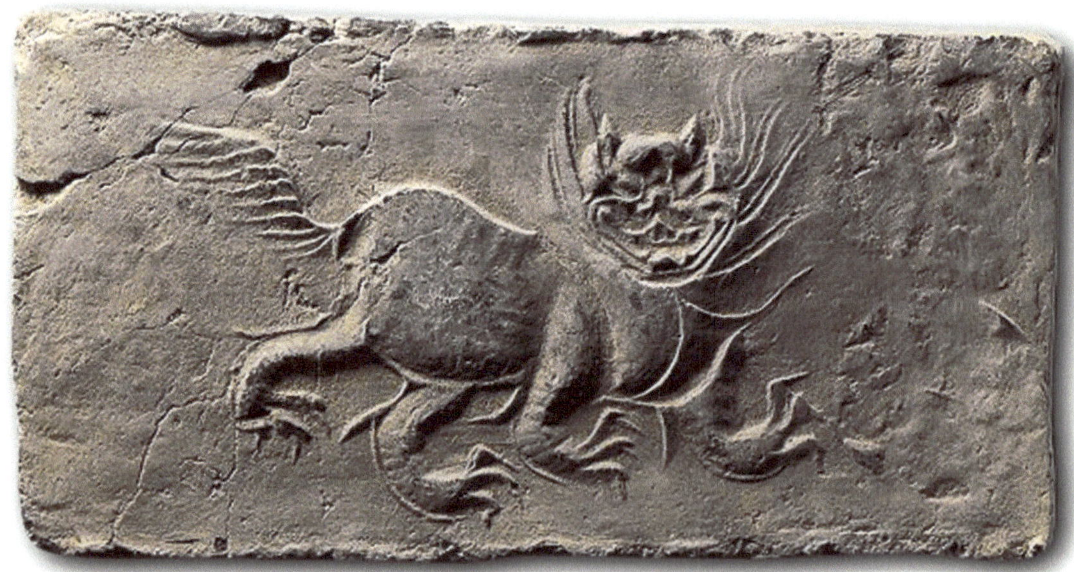

The most ancient Chinese metaphors for the primordial forces of *yang* and *yin* were the Blue Dragon (*qinglong*) and Unicorn (*qilin*) respectively. The images opposite are of clay tomb tiles excavated in 1988 at Jinqueshan. From the Eastern Han dynasty (25-220 CE) or later, they are now part of the collection of the Linyi Municipal Museum. Photos courtesy of the China Institute Gallery, New York.

FOREWORD

In the spring of 1993, I was invited to Fairfield, Iowa, to teach a *taiji* (t'ai chi) and *qigong* (ch'i kung) seminar. This was first seminar I gave after arriving in the USA in 1991. At that time, I spoke only broken English and came to meet this tall, gentle, soft-spoken man with a strong English accent. After the first handshake and greeting, we had felt a deep connection beyond language. Since then, we have become very close friends.

Max Wright has such a deep love and passion for *taiji*, and he also has such great respect for the tradition. Not only does he practice *taiji*, but he also spends a great deal of time in researching the essence of the art. I am very impressed with his learning ability and the knowledge he has of *taiji*.

I have seen many people practice *taiji*, but I have seen so few people genuinely learning the true *taiji*. Max has good teachers and always shows a hunger for new knowledge. His love and respect of *taiji* leads him toward the decoding of the *taiji* diagram today.

I always want to show the secrets of the *taiji* diagram to people who love the practice and philosophy. I am so glad that Max has done this also. He can speak "Chinese" better than me. It is so hard for me to convey the right nuance without using my own language. Max has made a great contribution to our *taiji* society.

In my *Wudang* tradition, *taiji* includes three concepts or disciplines. They are *Wu Ji, Tai Ji* and *Liang Yi.* The *Wu Ji* aspect prescribes meditation. From within the tranquility, stillness brings forth *yuan* (original) *qi*, transmuting *Jing* to *Qi*. After that you will need to practice *taiji* movement to balance and harmonize the *yin* and *yang qi* inside the energy system of the body. Finally, we can use the trained *yin* or *yang qi* in the practice of *Liang Yi* to demonstrate the different applications of *kung fu* form, such as *fajing*.

The simple *taiji* diagram portrays the entire process of creation as described by *Laozi* and developed through the internal martial arts. All elements of the progression are clearly shown in the diagram and you get a real sense of the dynamism in the process. Add the concept of *bagua* and you've got a complete picture of reality.

But Taoist literature is focused on secretly-couched alchemical practices. It's hard to unravel the process of creation from formulas to refine the *qi* in the human body. It's not scientific or general. Also, the historical explanation for the evolution of the *bagua* from *yin* and *yang* has a lot of limitation. Max shows that it follows the same evolution as expressed in the diagram.

Taiji is the concrete expression of the principles of the diagram. In this way, it takes something very subtle, very precious, and makes it plain to see on the surface of life.

The *taiji* diagram has the whole of Nature's secrets encoded into it. Meditation will make the process part of your conscious awareness. Bring this to the *taiji* form and you have a formula for fast growth to higher states of consciousness.

These principles of the diagram work in outside day-to-day life too. Max provides a framework to introduce a better *taiji*-based, consciousness-based approach to daily life.

It is my honor to write this foreword for Max. I hope to see more of his writing in the near future.

曾永祥

Tseng Yun-Xiang

Ft Collins, Colorado
November 4, 2006

[Master Yun Xiang Tseng was raised and trained in the famous Wu Dang temple in HuBei province. He is a 14th generation priest of the Zhang San Feng lineage, and 25th generation Dragon Gate branch (Longmen sect) lineage. His academy in the mountains of northern Colorado was authorized by the late Grandmaster Li Cheng Yu and established to bring to the USA the authentic Wu Dang Taoist teachings that have been passed on in an unbroken living tradition for 700 years. (www.wudangtao.net/ustemple)]

LOOKING INTO THE EYES OF NATURE

This work presents the chief insights of a lifetime practice in meditation and martial arts. It is a mystery to me why I should have been blessed with the patient guidance of so many extraordinarily talented teachers. I have had the good fortune to meet and train under several of the greatest masters of our age. The essence of what they imparted to me is blended together in this little book and, if it helps shed some light on Nature's greater mysteries, then perhaps I shall have repaid them in some measure. Here I would like to honor those most directly responsible for the advancement of my progress towards truly looking through the eyes of Nature...

I began Transcendental Meditation (TM) in Johannesburg, South Africa, in 1974—the same year that I was introduced to Japanese karate. As my practice of TM advanced, I was drawn more and more to the internal martial arts and especially t'ai chi. A big difference between my journey and that of a lot of my t'ai chi colleagues was that the inner experience of meditation led me to a deeper realization of the martial arts—not the other way around.

So the basis of my modest attainment is the practical and philosophical application of Vedic Science as brought to light and revived by His Holiness Maharishi Mahesh Yogi. To him I owe an enormous debt of gratitude. Ironically, I once heard Maharishi be quite disparaging about t'ai chi ch'uan as a tool for directly developing higher states of consciousness. It's been my reality check for over 20 years while I nevertheless explored it deeply. I do believe that with the basis of my study rooted in my understanding of his Vedic Science, I have not altogether wasted my time!

There were a number of bright beacons on my path.

Master Eddie Jardine, founder of the T'ai Chi Society of South Africa, accepted me as a t'ai chi student back in 1985. A teacher more capable, generous, modest and truly dedicated to his art you will not find. To Sifu I owe not only my abiding love of the t'ai chi form, but my appreciation for what is real in both practice and attitude.

Grandmaster Hsiung Wei, the living demonstration of what perfect t'ai chi looks like (and feels like to be on the receiving end), represents most clearly what I aspire to both inside and outside of the training room.

My friend Wudang Master Tseng Yun-Xiang—an accomplished martial artist and exceptionally gifted healer—was instrumental in helping me make all the connections between the t'ai chi form and what happens energetically and internally when the right attention is brought to the practice.

Finally, I would like to thank those great souls who acted as lenses to bring the world into better focus once I began to see: Shihan Mark Saito, Grandmaster Zhao Zeng-fu, and the late Grandmaster Duan Yu-chang.

This book was written to show how unbelievably complete the humble t'ai chi diagram —the well-known Yin-Yang fishes symbol - is in explaining the fundamental process of creation throughout the universe. The diagram shows us how each form evolves and changes, and its relationship with the eternal non-changing, the formless.

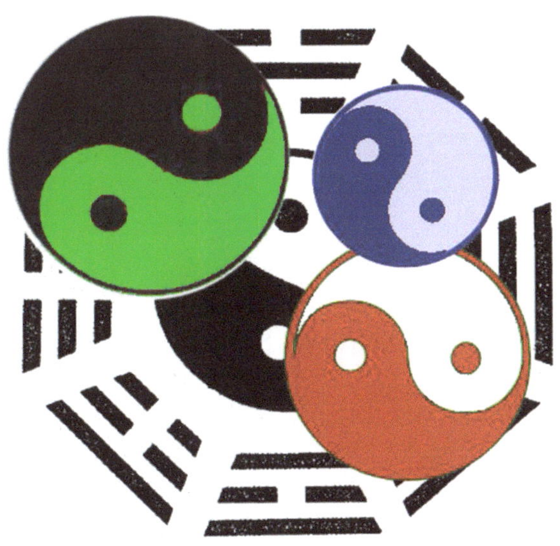

There will be no dry expositions of Vedic or Taoist scholarship, or complicated minutiae of inaccessible techniques about energy manipulation in these pages—I don't have the patience for them. I offer just the basic, intuitively obvious concepts needed to explain the diagram. I have subtitled the book: "A T'ai Chi Player's Guide to the Way Things Are." It's a practical manual for martial artists, meditators, business managers, and all other seekers who need to "get" it, but can't deal with New Age nirvana or arcane esoterica. It is not in my nature to speculate about something that hasn't been my personal experience.

I had difficulty deciding whether to call the book "Looking *Through* the Eyes of Nature" or "Looking *Into* the Eyes of Nature." Most of the information is intellectually looking into the process from the outside, but the goal is to develop our awareness, and so realize our intrinsic participation in the process—and that would be looking *through* the eyes of Nature. So I chose the first title to emphasize the ultimate purpose of the diagram in guiding us to experience the process firsthand.

When I was a child growing up in England, my mother firmly disapproved of American television. So I did not often get to watch the adventures of Hanna Barbera's cartoon character, Quick Draw McGraw. For those of you too young to have been watching television a decade before the first men set foot on the moon, Quick Draw McGraw was a hapless gun-slinging horse, the sheriff of an old Wild West town. In the opening credits, Quick Draw would find himself racing down the mountain on a stagecoach, with the bad guys in hot pursuit. There would be bullets flying everywhere and of course our hero would be stoically without any control of the situation whatsoever. As a kid, my favorite part was when the coach's axles would extend themselves—like doing the splits—so that the wheels could negotiate the sudden appearance in the road of ravines and such.

My journey through life has been a bit like those wheels. On the one side there was meditation with all its ancient Indian heritage and flavors. On the other, the essentially Taoist tradition of t'ai chi. Many times, when the inevitable bumps and potholes cropped up along the path, the axles of my practice had to stretch to accommodate the two, seemingly not always parallel, tracks. Moreover, the idea of a stagecoach careening down the mountainside under its own inertia and the force of gravity—with the horse *riding* it—is an interesting metaphor for how this reluctant seeker sped off down the road of life in spite of himself. With the help of the t'ai chi diagram (or t'ai chi tu), we'll see how the two paths are actually flawlessly parallel and how the one is the perfect commentary on the other.

There will be some Chinese names and terms scattered throughout the text. These days, with the growing influence of mainland China in the martial arts, the use of *pinyin* is becoming much more prevalent. But most lay people are still more familiar with the older Wade-Giles romanization—so this will be the standard with the *pinyin* italicized in parentheses. It will be necessary also to introduce a couple of Sanskrit terms, and these will be in bold italics.

I recently had something of an epiphany, the solution to a nagging puzzle that had vexed me for a very long time. And however obvious the explanation might have been to more learned initiates, in my mind the riddle held the key to the greatest mysteries. Arriving at this clarification after so many years was a great relief—and inspired me to write down my insights and musings. I will come to the problem later; what's important now is that it was the t'ai chi diagram that provided the answer.

Through the diagram, we will discover how the earthy common sense of the traditional Chinese world view can be enriched with the descriptive precision of the ancient Indian perspective. The diagram is a delicate compass to tell us where we are now and where we're going. It's just that the needle on this compass continually goes round and round—which it what it's supposed to do.

Whether you're searching for a beautiful liquid t'ai chi form, or hoping to enhance your meditation; whether your path is the explosive force of fa jing, or more peaceably understanding the mechanics of manifestation at every level of creation; whether you need a novel road map for explaining corporate office dynamics, or you're simply just looking to discover the path of least resistance through life, the exquisitely uncomplicated t'ai chi tu can be your window on the workings of Nature.

Max Wright
August, 2006
Fayetteville, Arkansas

ORIGIN OF THE DIAGRAM

Traditional martial arts, meditation practice, enlightenment, and life in general are all about being conscious. The t'ai chi diagram is an instruction manual for being conscious. Life is all about being present in the Now, the only moment that is real. Nonetheless, although there's nothing Zen about history, it will be useful to have an understanding of how the diagram has evolved over the last thousand years or so.

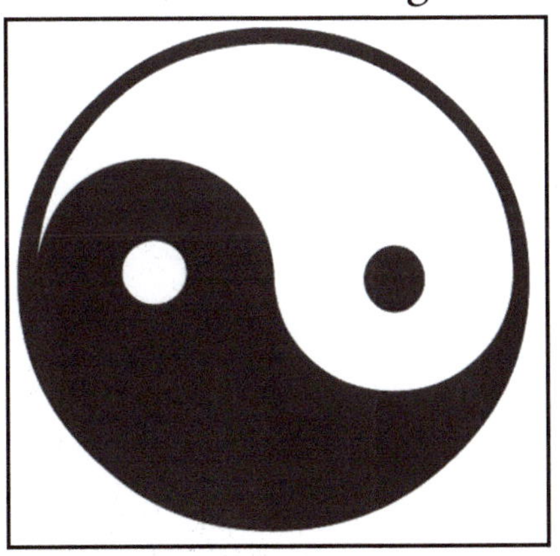

Here we see the modern Yin-Yang diagram with which everyone is familiar. I am afraid that it has fallen victim to oversimplification. Like the popular Yang-style t'ai chi ch'uan (*taijiquan*), it has been rendered completely innocuous to the casual observer—unless you already know what is buried within it. Although I have studied several styles of t'ai chi, my first and favorite is traditional Yang. The Yang form, and the diagram itself, both need a little research to uncover their secrets. However, this watered-down diagram is still a wonderful exposition of how our t'ai chi should flow on the surface from one posture to the next, and of how life cycles progress as a whole.

What is misleading about the contemporary picture on the previous page is the primary subject of this book—the anatomy of what Deepak Chopra calls "The Gap." Our concern is with the "eyes" in the diagram. What are they? What do they do? And how do they do it?

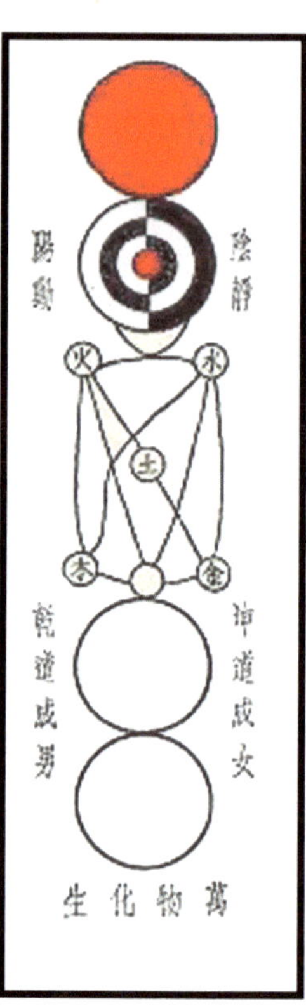

In ancient times, the diagram didn't even have the obvious "eyes" it has today.

The familiar yin-yang diagram, or t'ai chi tu (*taijitu*) evolved from the "Diagram of the Supreme Ultimate." This original layout (shown at right) is attributed to Chou Tun-I (*Zhou Dunyi*) who lived from 1017–1073 during the Song dynasty.

However, the Chou Tun-I version of the diagram has a much older heritage in that it is essentially a top-down re-reading of the alchemical "Diagram of the Infinite" passed down from the revered Taoist master Chen Tuan (906-989).

Over the centuries, the diagram was refined and simplified.

The beautiful Ming-era diagram on the next page is a woodblock print from 1623. Much more like our modern version, it forms a part of the "Compendium of Diagrams" by Zhang Huang. This image is reprinted by kind courtesy of The University of Chicago Library, East Asian collection.

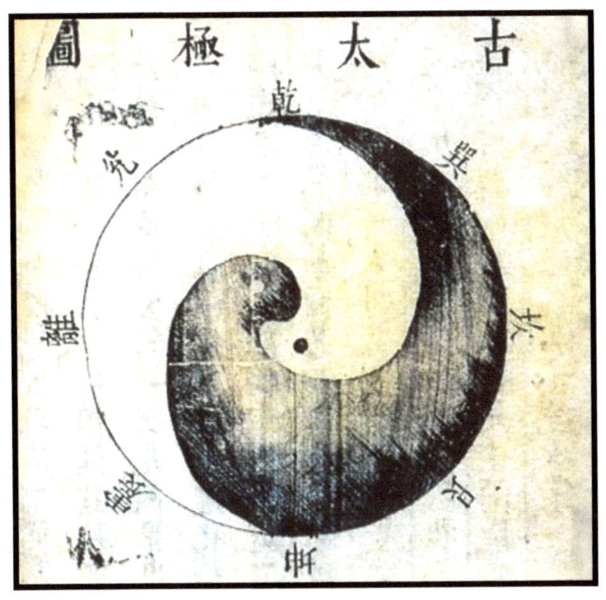

A concept of great importance in t'ai chi practice is what Professor Cheng Man-ching called "folding and plaiting". Folding is the essential secret of t'ai chi ch'uan and is the basis of an effective and beautiful performance, plus the root of emitting energy. It is also intimately related to the functioning of the "eyes" in the diagram. These things almost jump out of the old 17th century woodblock diagram—as we'll discuss later. In addition, when analyzing the mechanics from a Vedic Science perspective, many more "secrets" come to light using the older layout.

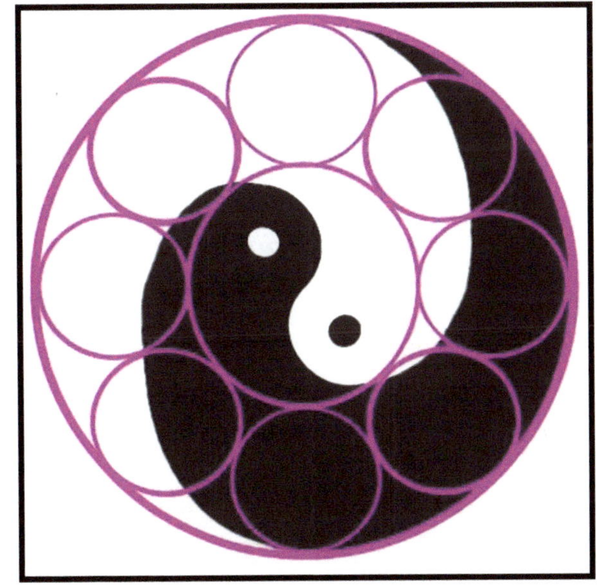

The core scripture of Vedic texts is the "Rig Veda". That work is commonly divided into ten books or ***mandalas*** (literally circles). Likewise, I have superimposed ten circles over the older-style diagram (right). There are eight smaller circles, plus a central circle, and an all-encompassing tenth circle around the whole thing. Note the modern t'ai chi symbol, self-contained within the central circle (***mandala 1***).

So the t'ai chi diagram is an exquisite

commentary on the workings of Nature. This new arrangement of the circles or **mandalas** over the basic diagram is pleasing from another point of view because it demonstrates perhaps the most pervasive blueprint of creation—the Golden Mean. The Golden Mean describes the way that things in nature are arranged, grow and evolve—it is Nature's signature. We find it in everything from the structure of DNA to leaf growth in plants to the relationships between the bodies of the solar system itself. The Golden Mean or Fibonacci number is seen in all natural systems, from the perfect spiraling of sea shells to the form of vast galaxies.

For clarity's sake, we have drawn the outer circle circumscribing the eight smaller circles so that it just touches their perimeters. However, if the outer circle or 10th **mandala** is drawn through the centers of the small **mandalas**, then the diagram displays *phi* —the Golden Mean constant of nature—at all levels. The relationship of the small circles to the inner 1st **mandala** delivers *phi* to an accuracy of 99.7%. The ratio is 1 to 1.613. The ratio of the inner **mandala 1** to the outer **mandala 10** again provides *phi* to an accuracy of 99.9%. This new ratio is 1.613 to 2.613.

[The actual mathematical value of *phi* to six decimal places is 1.618034. Apart from being displayed in every facet of nature, *phi* is a very intriguing number. It is the only quantity that when squared is equal to itself plus one (2.618). Similarly, if you divide *phi* into one you get *phi* minus one (0.618).]

This high degree of congruence between the t'ai chi diagram, the herald of traditional Chinese cosmology, plus the foundation of the "I-Ching" (as we will see later), together with the core classic of Vedic knowledge, the "Rig Veda", and now the manifest guiding principle of Nature's workings (the Golden Mean), gives us great confidence that our forthcoming analysis will illuminate many secrets of the world around us.

In subsequent chapters, we will use this new modified version to explain how the diagram relates to the evolution of the "I-Ching" (*Yijing* or "Book of Changes"), how the diagram is a commentary of the Taoist theory of manifestation and evolution laid out in Lao Tzu's "Tao Te Ching", and finally we will see how it can all be elucidated using the Vedic Science encapsulated within the "Rig Veda".

第四十二章　道化

道生一。一生二。二生三。三生萬物。萬物負陰而抱陽。冲氣以爲和。人之所惡。唯孤寡不穀。而王公以爲稱。故或損之而益。或益之而損。人之所教。我亦教之。强梁者。不得其死。吾將以爲教父。

THE ORIGIN OF EVERYTHING ELSE

The "Tao Te Ching" is the quintessential canonical text of Taoism, and the t'ai chi symbol is its coat of arms.

"Tao Te Ching" (*Dao De Jing*)

From stanza 42, **"Transformations of the Tao"**

The Tao gives birth to One.
One gives birth to Two.
Two gives birth to Three.
Three gives birth to the ten thousand things.

Lao Tzu (*Laozi*—6th century BCE)

It is precisely this process of creation that the t'ai chi diagram portrays so elegantly. But what does it mean? Both Lao Tzu and the diagram suggest a progression from One to Two, from Two to Three, and from there everything else.

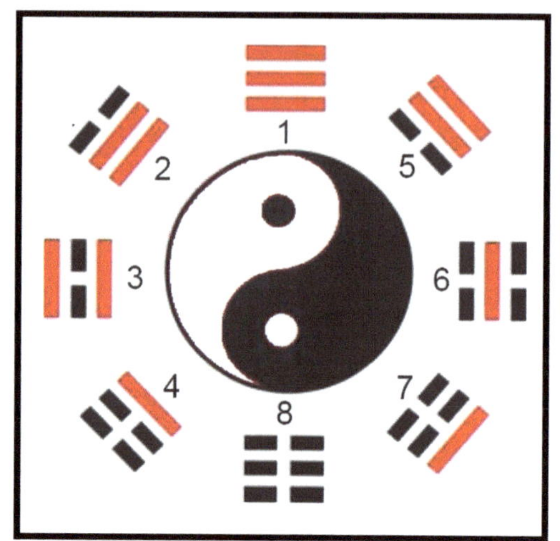

The t'ai chi diagram is frequently associated with the traditional eight-sided *bagua* (or the I-Ching trigrams), and both are used to describe the world in general and martial arts postures in particular. We'll elaborate upon the *bagua* later, but for now I'll remark that in every analysis of the subject that I have studied, the evolution of the trigrams is shown in terms of One to Two, Two to Four, Four to Eight, and from there everything else.

So which progression is it? Is it from One to Two to Three to everything? Or is it from One to Two to Four to Eight to everything? If there are inconsistencies in the bedrock foundation, what are we to believe of the philosophical edifices and martial arts explanations that are built upon them? By taking recourse to a brief overview of the principal Vedic classic called "Rig Veda", we will be able to clarify Lao Tzu and, at the same time, demonstrate a more credible basis for the origination of the *bagua* trigrams. First, let's go over the principal elements that make up the t'ai chi diagram…

i) The background is a plain white, unadorned circle. This represents wu chi (*wuji*), the unmanifest source of all relative creation. This is the One referred to in Lao Tzu.

ii) Superimposed upon wu chi are the black (*yin*) and white (*yang*) "fishes" that eternally mutate into one another. These are the Two.

iii) The third element of the t'ai chi diagram is the wavy line, curving back on itself, that separates the yin and yang portions. This symbolizes the dynamic interface between yin and yang. In this way, we have the idea of the yin quality, the yang quality, and the relationship between them—the Three. As we will see further on, these Three form the basis of the trigrams—which can be combined together to explain everything (the "ten thousand things").

iv) The final elements are the "eyes"—but we're not going to examine them until a little later when we deal with the Gap.

The philosophical systems of ancient Vedic India and Taoist China (and incidentally, also modern theoretical physics) each explain the mechanics of relative manifestation as a process of sequential symmetry breaking from out of a primordial undifferentiated wholeness. The world's cultures all describe this original singularity as omniscient, omnipresent and omnipotent. Society has many names for it: Being, Pure Consciousness, God (the impersonal aspect), the vacuum state of the quantum field, the Unified Field of all the Laws of Nature, etc. We have noted that in traditional Chinese thought, it is known as wu chi (*wuji*), and is symbolized by an empty white circle. Beyond space, time and causation, it is impossible to describe it in relative terms —it just is. This is self-evident, and it's also obviously not inert. It is conscious, it is aware. Therefore, about the only characteristics that can be ascribed to it are existence and intelligence (or pure awareness). The Existence aspect is primordial *yang* and the Intelligence aspect is primordial *yin*. Thus the One can be conceived of as Two. According to Vedic Science, when primordial existence becomes conscious, and primordial intelligence becomes intelligent, then the dynamism of creative intelligence brings forth from unity the entire abundance of diversity.

Before manifest creation emerges, wu chi (the primordial source) is aware only of itself. However, being conscious of itself produces the idea of movement. There is a curving or folding back in the process of wu chi becoming aware of itself—which in turn creates a sort of unmanifest pre-geometry. The dynamism of becoming Self-aware creates a virtual space/time continuum, the original template for the mechanics of differentiation. Out of the One comes the idea of the Three—wu chi expressed as the knower or subject (wu chi, itself), the known or object (itself), and the process of knowing (also itself, by its own inherent nature).

This is the essential 3-in-1 nature of the universe and is the symbolism of the famous t'ai chi diagram, where the duality of yin and yang perpetually transmute into each other (wholeness of the circle divided into yin, yang, and mutual dynamism). It is Three, but it is really One.

Now we're going to switch to the Vedic Science of India perspective to analyze Lao Tzu's words. In order to do that, we need to introduce a few Sanskrit terms.

The Vedic terminology for the undifferentiated wu chi is ***samhita*** (wholeness or singularity, pronounced sung-yee-tuh)—which is composed of the three aspects: ***rishi***, ***devata*** and ***chhandas***. The concept of the knower is called ***rishi***, the dynamism aspect or process is called ***devata***, and the object of knowledge or known is ***chhandas***.

This idea of consciousness curving back upon itself is expressed in the first syllable of the first word, of the first verse, of the first book (or ***mandala***) of "Rig Veda". Each subsequent word and space, verse and chapter is an elaboration of the one before. Thus the whole story of creation through sequential differentiation evolves out of this very first expression of "Rig Veda". Maharishi has shown that the whole text is a commentary upon itself, perfect in its completeness and mathematical symmetry—but to see how the t'ai chi tu works, all we need consider is that first syllable: ***ak*** (from the first word ***Agnim***).

The original singularity (***samhita***) is the totality of all that is. So at the same time, it is both infinitely large and infinitesimally small. From the point of view of relativity in time and space, it's both here and there simultaneously.

In terms of the human voice, the sound where the mouth and throat (organs of speech) are most open is "ah." Conversely, a complete glottal stop ("gk") is the most fully closed configuration. Thus the first syllable of "Rig Veda" takes the reciter from the fullest expression of speech down to silence—and mirrors the process of the collapse of infinity onto its point value. This is the curving back progression of infinity knowing itself. Infinity, point value, and the dynamism of collapse. Knower, known and process of knowing. ***Rishi***, ***Chhandas***, and ***Devata*** (process).

To summarize, we have gone from One (singularity/***samhita***/wu-chi), to Two (existence/yang and intelligence/yin), to Three (knower, process and known/***rishi, devata*** and ***chhandas***/t'ai-chi). This process is illustrated by the t'ai chi symbol that displays the dynamical relationship between the primordial forces that shape the universe.

Whatever our cultural background, tradition ties our source back to some form of trinity: The Three Pure Ones of Taoism; Father, Son and Holy Ghost of Christianity; Brahma, Vishnu and Shiva of Hinduism; Hilbert Space, Operators and States of Theoretical Physics; Heaven, Earth and Man…

The collapse of consciousness from infinitely expanded to its point value happens with infinite frequency, giving rise to the "cosmic hum". In the following section, we will see how the trinity somersaulting upon itself gives rise to the whole multiplicity of relative creation (Lao Tzu's "ten thousand things").

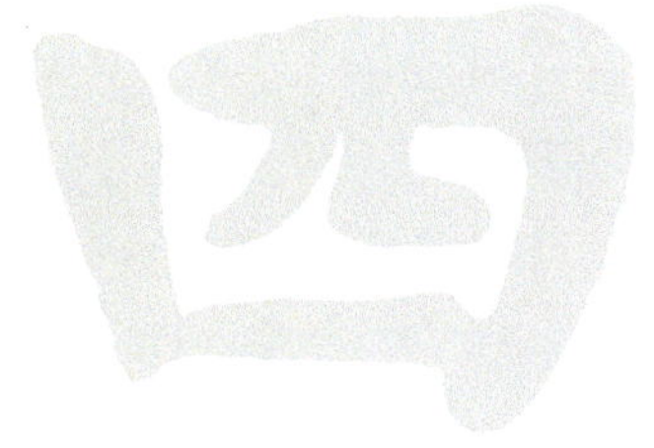

3-IN-1

Here in the "real" world of our senses, we tend to see and experience things only in terms of objectivity—the observer, the observed, and the process of observing—and we miss the fundamental unity of it all. It is said that the root cause of human suffering is in our failure to perceive that our fascination with the mirage of the Three prevents us from cognizing the One. In ancient scripture, this is called the mistake of the intellect (***pragya-aparadha***).

The universe, and any part of it, is the co-existence of two perspectives. It is One and Three at the same time. Three and One. Always. In any living system, from the smallest amoeba to a corporate enterprise and beyond, nested within each unit there is always the expression of Three. Harmony (balance) comes from perception and experience of the One, and success comes from understanding and managing the roles of and relationships between the Three.

Relative creation comes about by the self-referral, self-interacting play of the Three with one another in the field of the One. Looking at the t'ai chi diagram, the yin and yang "fishes" seem to be continuously somersaulting over each other. It is this infinite dynamism of the one value collapsing into its complement that creates the underlying vibration that gives rise to the manifest universe by sequential differentiation. We will see later that by initiating action at this pre-manifest level of reality, in the gap or space between collapses, we can specify or influence the outcome of a situation in the outside world of our day to day senses.

With our two previously described characteristics of unmanifest pure Being (the One), namely existence (*yang*) and intelligence (*yin*), we essentially have a binary system (the Two). This duality could be looked at in terms of infinitely large and infinitely small, or light and dark, masculine and feminine, and so on—but I prefer our original descriptions of primordial latencies or ideas within the formless transcendental field.

When we cast these two primordial qualities across three dimensions (knower/***rishi***, process/***devata*** and known/***chhandas***—which constitute the Three), we arrive at eight primary transformations of creative intelligence ($2^3 = 8$). These "transformations of creative intelligence" spring forth from the gaps between collapses of impulses of creative intelligence, and are the "Transformations of the Tao"—the title of the 42nd stanza of Lao Tzu that we looked at in the previous chapter.

In the oral tradition of "Rig Veda", this is represented by the sounds of the syllables and the silence of the gaps between them. Thus "ak," the first syllable in "Rig Veda", collapses in eight modalities from "ah" into its point value, "gk." Vedic terminology for these eight foundational characteristics (or natures) is ***prakritis***. The rest of the first ***mandala*** (or book) of "Rig Veda" is the elaboration of the sequential unfoldment of these eight natures from the collapse of wholeness. Each of the eight ***prakritis*** is analyzed in terms of ***rishi, devata and chhandas***. Then each of these is further expounded, one verse for each in terms of each of the 8 modalities, i.e. 24 x 8 for a total of 192 verses. Or, looking at it from another angle, 64 possibilities of manifestation, each viewed through its relationship with ***rishi*** (knower), ***devata*** (process of knowing), and ***chhandas*** (known), i.e. 64 x 3 for a total of 192 expressions.

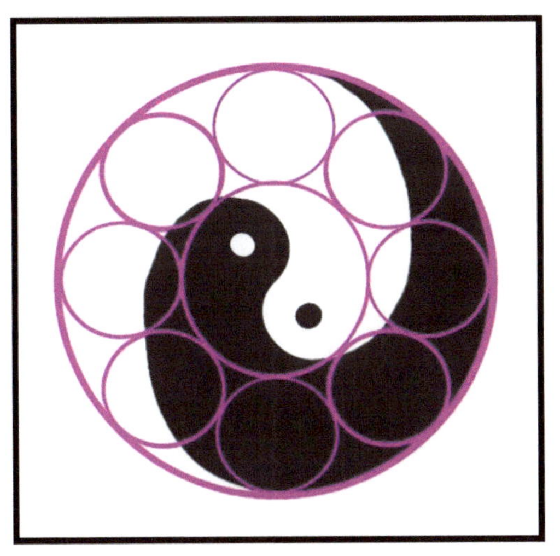

Remember that "Rig Veda" consists of 10 ***mandalas***, the most important of which are the first – which describes the self-referral mechanics of creation—and the tenth, whose 192 verses tie it all together as a commentary on the 192 gaps between the verses of the first ***mandala***. ***Mandalas*** two through nine serve as a commentary on each of the eight prakritis.

Those readers familiar with Chinese classical literature and the "I-Ching" (*Yijing* or "Book of Changes"), but who have not previously been exposed to the rudiments of Vedic Science, must be jumping up and down with excitement over the connections they're making…

In ancient China, the matriarchal elders of the Fu Hsi clan somehow also determined that there were eight fundamental qualities or natures (*ba gua*) to relative creation. They expressed these building blocks as sets of three lines (trigrams), each describing a particular configuration of *yin* (broken lines) and *yang* (solid lines). The lines represented heaven (knower), earth (known) and man (the dynamic pivot in the central place). Each trigram displays an aspect of the mutual inter-relationships of the observer/knower, observed/known and dynamism/process features of the pre-manifest wholeness.

They are thus the condensation of all possible basic interactions between the elements of the t'ai chi. Of course, the legendary King Wen then combined each trigram with each possible combination of other trigram, yielding 64 hexagrams that described all the basic conditions of relative existence. And so the "I-Ching" was born.

And while we're at it: In terms of the superstring models of modern theoretical physics, the observer quality is represented by Hilbert Space, the dynamism quality by the Operators, and the observed aspect corresponds to States. In addition to the purely bosonic modes associated with the abstract space-time arena in which the string moves, the mathematics reveals precisely eight fundamental fermionic degrees of freedom intrinsic to the string itself. Once again, all of creation springs forth by sequential symmetry breaking. Through the collapse of the wave function, virtual fluctuations in the quantum field precipitate out as the particles and their interactions that make up concrete experience. Previously we overlaid the old version t'ai chi diagram with 10 circles representing the ***mandalas***. Now, armed with this new insight from "Rig Veda", let's look at our modified t'ai chi diagram once more, adding in the evolution of the trigrams and associated ***mandala*** numbers.

The trigrams are read from bottom to top, and when arranged in this ***mandala*** format, start at the line closest to the center.

Any trigram can transmute into any other simply by the transformation of any of the component lines into its polar opposite. This process is the collapse of a *yang* impulse into a *yin* impulse, and vice versa, which happens in the gap.

Although some learned sinologists have said the opposite, it makes more sense to read the trigrams with the Heaven (knower) line at the bottom, followed by Man (the process or dynamism aspect) in the center, and finally Earth (the known or objective value) at the top. In this way the progression of trigram evolution around the *bagua* is more intuitively satisfying.

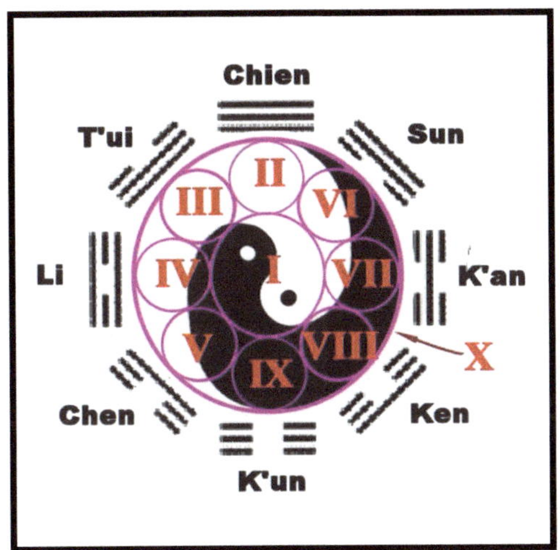

The accepted order of the trigrams follows the order given for the mandalas—that is, from Chien through to Chen, and then from Sun around to K'un. These are the feelings that I get from the structure of the eight trigrams:

Chien (*qian*) means "heaven" and signifies power and creativity. All the aspects of knower (***rishi***/heaven), process (***devata***/man), and known (***chhandas***/earth) are fully expressed as solid (*yang*) lines.

T'ui (*dui*) means "lake" or "marsh" and has the connotation of pleasure and satisfaction. The subject/knower and dynamism values are being expressed.

Li suggests "fire" with a sense of suddenness, as in lightning or the sun. Li signifies brightness and beauty. There is the *yang* quality expressed on the outside, but yielding to change through transformation within.

Chen (*zhen*) means "thunder." The trigram consists of passive, quiescent lines—but with a strong yang line in the first place, producing the idea of initiating movement or excitement.

Sun (*xun*) is "wind" or "wood", with strong lines except for the subject/rishi quality, connoting flexibility and penetration.

K'an means "water" in the sense of flowing swiftly—as in a stream or through a gorge. The trigram shows yielding softness on the outside, but strength within. This gives the feeling of change, difficulty or danger.

Ken (*gen*) means "mountain" and connotes that which arrests movement or progress. The object/***chhandas*** quality is strong, but there is no motivation in the other lines to shift the inertia.

K'un is "earth" where all lines are yin and yielding, conveying the idea of passivity, submissiveness, nourishment and receptivity.

Going back to the vantage of Vedic Science, the "Rig Veda" concerns itself with ultimate reality as it expresses itself through the human nervous system. We have discussed the first word of the first ***mandala*** of the text as being "Agnim". ***Agni*** is the *yang*, bright, fiery aspect of consciousness. Its polar opposite is ***Soma***, the *yin*, cohesive, nourishing principle in the universe. ***Indra*** is the lively manifestation of consciousness, ***Agni***, in the human physiology. Many are the paths, functions and faculties that streams of awakened consciousness condense into, but they all arise from ***Agni***, blazing up the spine as ***Indra***.

It is highly revealing to look at the devata (deity or animating principle) attributed to the hymns of each ***mandala***. Watch the way the hymns are addressed, and how this changes with the proportion of *yin* and *yang* and the ***mandalas'*** progress around the *bagua* in the traditionally prescribed order:

Mandala #1 (***Agni Mandala***), in the center of the diagram, concerns the mechanics of creation—how fullness of "ah" collapses to its point value of "gk." This is the story of the lively field of all possibilities, the story of the Gap. All verses are addressed to ***Agni***.

Mandala #2 corresponds to the Chien trigram (fully *yang*) and the ***devata*** is mainly

Agni and ***Indra***. This position in the *bagua* is associated with an "eye" and marks the greatest *yang* potential in the diagram. As we'll see later, the collapse of this expression of creative intelligence (the Tao) gives rise to the fabled Taoist elixir of immortality, to ***soma*** the nectar of the gods. It is as though this room had a secret passage leading directly to the *yin* part of the mansion.

Mandala #3 is predominately *yang*, occupying the place of the trigram T'ui. Once again, this ***mandala*** has most of its verses dedicated to ***Agni*** and ***Indra***.

Mandala #4 corresponds to Li—which is a cardinal trigram and predominately *yang*. The hymns in this ***mandala*** are also mainly addressed to ***Agni*** and ***Indra***.

Mandala #5 occupies the position of the fourth trigram called Chen. This trigram is at the very start of the *yang* cycle and is still predominately *yin*. Hymns in this mandala are addressed to ***Agni*** and ***Indra***, but also to various other deities. Two of the hymns are to the dawn—an appealing metaphor for the beginning of the bright *yang* evolution.

Mandala #6 is associated with Sun, the fifth trigram and the start of the *yin* cycle. This trigram is mostly *yang* with a glimmer of young *yin*. Again we find the hymns addressed predominately to ***Agni*** and ***Indra***.

Mandala #7 is at the *yin* cardinal point of change, K'an. There are many deities mentioned in this ***mandala*** including the fountainhead, ***Agni*** and ***Indra***.

Mandala #8 corresponds to Ken, an almost entirely *yin* trigram. The hymns in this book are addressed to many different deities.

Mandala #9 (***Soma Mandala***) is in K'un, the completely *yin* position. The sole deity, except for parts of just three hymns in this book, is ***soma pavamana***. Another "eye" location, this position in the diagram corresponds to the point of greatest *yin* potential.

The start and culmination of the cycle, through its collapse gives rise to those more advanced experiences of ***Agni***—such as ***Kundalini***.

Mandala #10 is the wholeness, the aggregation and fulfillment of all the previous eight ***mandalas***. It is the reflection and commentary of the first ***mandala*** in the center. This final book is addressed to ***Agni*** plus the other deities. We have shown it as the all-encompassing circle around the t'ai chi diagram—the collective expression of the individual mechanics of evolution in the central place. It takes us from the personal to the societal arena. The deity of the first stanza of the final hymn is ***Agni***, and the remaining stanzas of that final hymn are addressed to ***Samjnana*** (the assembly). The actual sounds of the verses—the sounds of Nature talking about itself—are themselves the structural commentary (rather than their meaning in native Sanskrit or any other language). Yet even in English translation, the collective idea is maintained. The ***mandala*** ends with:

"Common be your intention; common be the wishes of your hearts; common be your thoughts, so that there may be thorough union among you."

So we find a high level of congruence between the Vedic and Taoist approaches to the internal workings of Nature. We have seen how relative creation springs from the self-referral dynamics of unchanging, undifferentiated wholeness (wu chi, ***samhita***). We have seen how manifestation arises through spontaneous sequential symmetry breaking, to give rise to eight primordial natures (*bagua*, ***prakritis***). In turn, the relationships between these eight qualities give rise to the 64 fundamental descriptions of relative existence codified in the hexagrams of the "I-Ching" (*Yijing*)—which in "Rig Veda" are further examined from the perspective of the knower (***rishi***), process of knowing (***devata***) or known (***chhandas***).

In addition, the t'ai chi diagram provides a clear tool to visualize how the various bagua transform into one another and progress to their points of maximum expression (Chien and K'un)—where we can directly access the Gap (the "eyes"). We will see how consciously accessing the Gap leads to personal evolution and growth towards experiences of higher states of consciousness and, how in turn, this provides the basis for productive societal relationships—the foundation for happy community and world peace.

[Note: "Rig Veda" was first committed to writing about the time that Chou Tun-I was formalizing the t'ai chi diagram. Until recently, the first and tenth ***mandalas*** were always shown to each have 191 ***suktas*** (verses or hymns)—not the 192 described above. But we must recall that "Rig Veda" has always been transmitted orally, and now Maharishi has demonstrated that the 97th verse is a silent ***sukta***. For this reason it was missed, and therefore not previously recorded in any written compilation.]

五

THE GAP

Self-defense techniques range from the sublime, through the subtle, to the ridiculous.

The ridiculous end of the spectrum is characterized by straight-line hard force-on-force attacks and defensive maneuvers. Western pugilistics would be a primitive example, as the philosophy is summed up by sayings such as: "The best form of defense is a resounding attack." Whatever the justifying motivation for the conflict, the outcome is always misfortune and compromise for at least one of the parties involved.

The subtle is characterized by the internal styles of martial arts like t'ai chi. Here the curved is emphasized over the straight, and softness and yielding over hard, direct force. Through a conscious understanding of the existence of the Gap, the opponent's own attacking energy is amplified and used to overwhelm him. Sifu Eddie Jardine, my teacher in South Africa, would say: "The best form of defense is to not be there when the attack arrives." Still, the field of conflict resolution is objective reality and success is obtained through the damage or discomfiture of the opposing party.

The sublime invokes the field effect in consciousness to disallow the birth of an enemy in the first place. This ultimate form of defense is explained by sayings such as this from the Yoga Sutras of Patanjali: "***Heyam duhkham anagatam*** (Avert the danger that has not yet come)." The whole situation is handled on the level of subjective reality, and resolution confers increase in the quality of life for all those involved. This is not at all the same as heroic tales of winning a war without shedding a drop of blood. The Gap-based methodology consists of engineering the underlying fabric of creation to produce a desired outcome that is life-supporting for everyone—not the manipulation of would-be protagonists through fear or other coercion.

The essential difference in these various approaches to defense lies in the skill of the practitioner to harness the power of the Gap.

Experts in the hard external techniques of martial arts rely on a fine understanding of the physics and structure of the physiology. Enormous athletic skill is involved. Using balance, leverage and timing, an energetic collapse on the gross physical level can be achieved that discharges a great amount of force. This explosive discharge from the Gap is called *fa li* (or emitting strength). The concept of ch'i (*qi*) is recognized, but it is in terms of hardness—like some kind of "Star Wars" force shield. An opponent is overcome by strength, dexterity, effort, and raw application of violent intention.

In contrast, experts in the internal styles concern themselves with training and accumulating energy at a more subtle level of Nature's functioning. Athleticism is not a prerequisite, but many years development in internal control is needed. Ch'i (*qi*) is understood as a supple whip-like resource, and utilized as the primary weapon. Duan Sifu used to say that the fingers are just the reconnaissance unit, the big guns are in the *dan tien* (belly energy reservoir). The t'ai chi classics tell us that the mind moves the ch'i, and the ch'i moves the body. So a more refined intention is applied at this level of technology. Although the effects can be equally devastating, the internal styles are less obviously violent. When an accomplished t'ai chi player finds the Gap and uses the collapse of attention to marshal and expel ch'i, it is called fa ching (*fajing*—emitting energy). In this case, an attack is like a needle buried within a soft silk cocoon, or an irresistible wave of the ocean that smothers or sweeps away all before it. The effect on the opponent is more potent, but less effort is expended by the practitioner.

Finally, experts in the Vedic technology of absolute defense concern themselves with exploring and manipulating consciousness directly from within the Gap. A simple fact of life is that progressively subtler levels of Nature's functioning are associated with greatly increased availability of energy. So working with the infinite organizing power of Nature itself results in invincible defense—with the expenditure of no effort whatsoever. Do less and accomplish more—this is the supreme efficiency of Nature. This is the power of the Gap.

After two decades of research and application, I am firmly convinced that the mindful discipline of t'ai chi ch'uan, in conjunction with a suitable meditation procedure to familiarize the practitioner with the experience of the transcendental field in which the Gap resides, is a highly effective way to develop the skills in consciousness required for the supreme value of martial arts: invincible defense without war or conflict.

In previous chapters, we saw that the Gap is Nature's mechanism for transforming all aspects of the ever-changing and evolving universe. This is true at all scales of existence.

For example, if an electron is traveling in one direction, but is needed for some reaction to be propagating in the opposite direction, then the first configuration briefly dissolves back into the quantum foam, as a new particle re-emerges in the required configuration. The electron winked out of existence into the Gap and then precipitated out again in the modality required to fulfill its purpose.

At the quantum mechanical level, events are influenced by the mere act of measuring them (Heisenberg). In other words, the application of our conscious attention, our consciousness, can alter the manifested results of random fluctuations in the underlying quantum field. Our directed attention at the subtlest strata of objective reality, the boundary zone between manifest and unmanifest, materially affects the physical outcome on the surface level of life.

Using the symbolism of the *bagua* trigrams, a simple flip of the yin or yang state of any of the ***rishi, devata or chhandas*** qualities in any of the eight constituent ***prakritis*** (natures), results in transformation to another configuration.

Consistent proactive management of our lives and environment can only be realized by having recourse to the Gap. The most astonishing feature of the human nervous system, available nowhere else in the known universe, is that it not only has the ability to perceive events on the quantum mechanical plane, but that it can consciously work below Planck scales—and indeed directly experience the ineffable, the Tao or unmanifested field of pure consciousness.

This is scientifically validated, not a matter of speculation. And if you've ever had a clear experience of transcendence during meditation or moments of inspiration, or been on the business end of the "magic" of a real t'ai chi master, then you know it to be true.

It isn't the purpose of this book to delve deeply into quantum cosmology, the physics and chemistry of dissipative structures, or even the technicalities of inner growth through meditation or martial arts. For that, the universe provides us with the teachers we need. We're just looking at how the t'ai chi diagram provides road markers and clear pointers along the way. The word Tao literally means "road" or "way". Whatever our chosen path, the formula for achievement is to safely and positively co-opt the intrinsic evolutionary power of Nature—located on the level of the Gap. The trick is to take a shortcut through the automatic cyclic rhythm of Nature and the t'ai chi diagram, and use the "eyes" to zip down the secret passage into the Gap.

There are four stages in the process of transformation or evolution:

- i) initial condition going into the Gap;
- ii) the silence of the Gap itself;
- iii) what is initiated in the Gap; and
- iv) the results brought out of the Gap.

To illustrate what happens in the "eyes" of the t'ai chi diagram, I will relate the "Problem of the Ardhanarishvara."

The word ***Ardhanarishvara*** comes from the Sanskrit meaning "Lord who is half woman." Like the t'ai chi diagram, the painting on the next page shows the totality of Nature as the coexistence of yang and yin aspects. We see the conjoined form of Lord Shiva (the father figure of the Hindu trinity) and His feminine counterpart, the goddess Durga (or Shakti).

The "problem" arises when we realize that ***Shiva***, the male, all-powerful figure is shown for all the world like the embodiment of *yin*. Look at the ash-colored skin, the cool

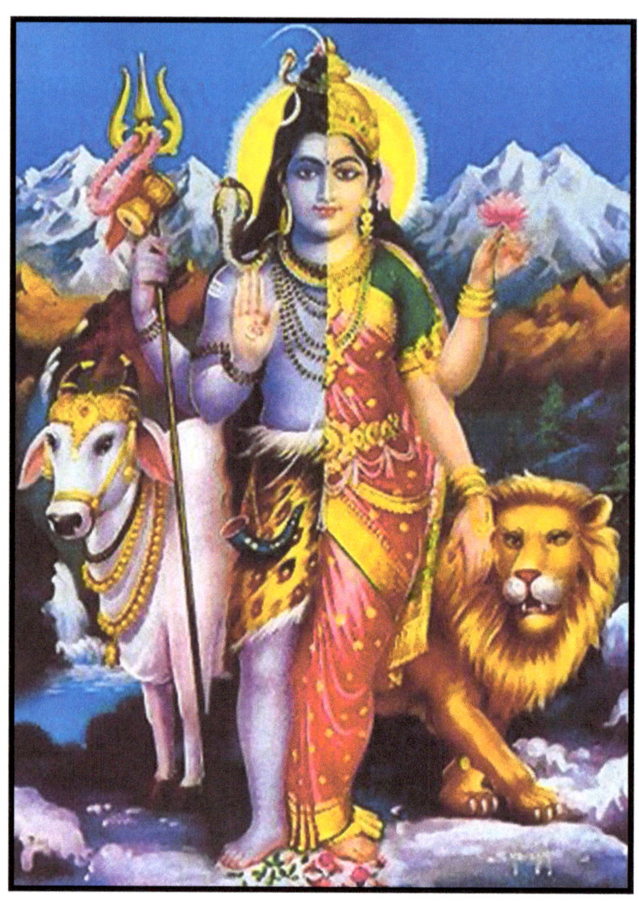

colors, the bull, the crescent moon, and so forth. Likewise, ***Shakti***, or the female principle, is presented in bright, warm *yang* colors and surroundings, and in the company of a golden lion.

This is how each of the deities of the picture is painted—even when they're the sole subject of an image. Moreover, there are all kinds of reasons traditionally attributed to the colors and context of each item associated with both ***Shiva*** and ***Shakti***.

Nonetheless, it seemed to me that there was an additional truth buried in the symbolism that I could not find explained in any literature or commentary that has crossed my desk.

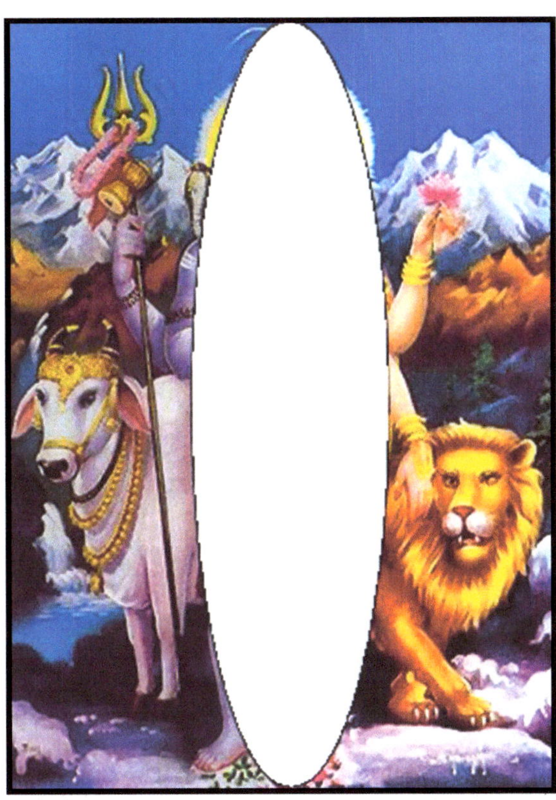

In this copy of the painting, I have masked out the primary subjects, ***Shiva*** and ***Durga*** (and I must admit, enhanced the contrast a little to emphasize my point). We can see that the right-hand side is the epitome of *yang*-ness, and conversely, the left half is pure *yin*.

When *yang* reaches its peak, it collapses into its point value (the "eye") and emerges from the Gap as *yin*. I locate ***Shiva*** in the upper *dan tien* in the crown of the head. It is this collapse that expresses the ***soma*** (Veda) or Taoist elixir—which then drops back down resounding into the lower *dan tien* (energy field) via the Regulating Channel. The Regulating Channel is the ch'i meridian (or energy pathway shown in blue below) connecting the tip of the tongue past the lower abdominal *dan tien* into the perineum.

Reciprocally, when *yin* reaches critical mass, it collapses into its complementary *yang* value (the bright "eye" in the K'un area of the t'ai chi diagram). I find ***Durga*** residing in the ocean of the lower *dan tien*, and Her collapse generates the ***Agni*** (lively *jing*) that travels through the Governing Vessel (red) from the perineum up the spinal column through the upper *dan tien* in the head, down to the roof of the mouth.

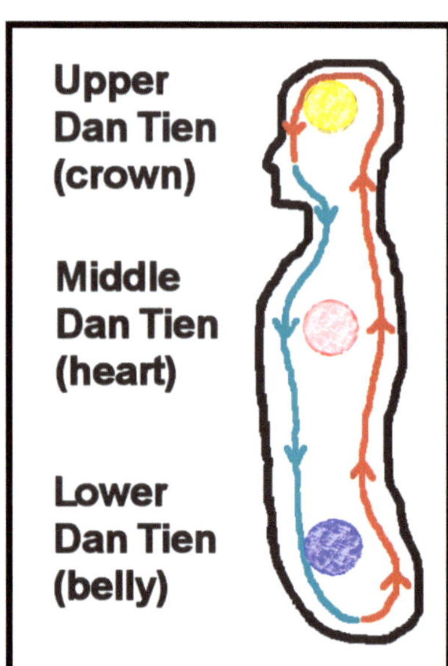

This is why ***Shiva*** is lord of transformation, and hailed as beneficent destroyer. And why His inseparable consort, ***Shakti***, is literally the source of creative (*yang*) energy.

Thus is the mystery resolved, and we discover ***Ardhavarishvara*** to be a beautiful commentary on the mechanics of manifestation of creative intelligence through the collapse of pure existence (primordial *yang*) onto its point value—which turns out to be pure intelligence (primordial *yin*)—which too evolves to its limit and then collapses to its *yang* point value, and so on.

In the foregoing analysis, we quietly glossed over the fact that the two primary energy channels or meridians don't exactly start and stop at their controlling *dan tien* fields. This will be our final analysis of the structure of the t'ai chi diagram before we move onto some practical applications of the knowledge.

My wife, Teresa Teravainen, is a practitioner in the profoundly subtle, yet deeply effective therapeutic healing modality known as TTouch (or Tellington Touch, after founder Linda Tellington-Jones). TTouch spontaneously enlivens the inherent intelligence of the body at the cellular level. This is effected by light, predominately circular strokes to the skin surface. The circles, however, continue around for a circle-and-a-quarter. You can try this yourself: If you're right-handed, gently massage the back of your left hand with the first two finger tips of your right hand. Move the skin round in a small 360 degree circle. If you listen to the sensation, you will find that it doesn't feel complete—not quite comfortable. Now go round in a circle from 12 o'clock, all the way around, and continue further through to three o'clock. A full circle-and-a-quarter. Does this feel better?

Similarly, in our older-version t'ai chi diagram – and this is what sets it apart from the modern styling—the *yang* and *yin* glyphs spiral around a bit further than their maximum values before collapsing into the "eyes".

And in the meridian system of the body, the Governing Vessel extends a little past the crown energy center down to the root of the nose. We connect it to the Regulating Vessel by placing the tip of our tongue onto the roof of the mouth. That meridian then extends down to the *dan tien*, and a little way past—down into the perineum, where it rejoins the Governing Vessel to pass through the base of the coccyx.

I don't know why this should be so. It just is and consequently feels right. And this is the practical secret of the Gap, of folding and plaiting in the t'ai chi form that we'll discuss in the next chapter.

There are specific prescriptions, conditions and prerequisites for exercising your skills in the Gap. Anything that can make this most mysterious of processes plain to see and validate will be a truly wonderful gift. T'ai chi ch'uan (*taijiquan*) is just such a gift.

六

T'AI CHI CH'UAN

As a welcome respite to all the theory, we're going to keep this chapter anecdotal. In the grand scheme of things, I could perhaps be called a good beginner—so I can't imagine foisting myself, uninvited, into my readers' t'ai chi practice. Perhaps the points can be made with a few stories…

For a number of years, I ran a flourishing t'ai chi club out of the small southeast Iowa town of Fairfield—at least until my bill-paying information-processing alter ego relocated me back to Long Island, New York.

Fairfield is home to Maharishi University of Management, where some of the world's most extensive ongoing experiments and demonstrations of the field effects of group consciousness have been successfully undertaken. But although Fairfield has less than 10,000 residents, it has a big heart in its own right and is a very unique community. It's like some sort of cosmic rendezvous, a hub on the network where all kinds of special souls from all over the globe drop in to visit. Similarly, my school was a closely knit group and a very happy place—and the most amazing martial arts luminaries from across the country just used to wander in. Occasionally we'd invite a guest teacher, but the best ones just showed up on the doorstep. It's important to have a special place to focus and sustain the energies of your journey. The International T'ai Chi Society of Fairfield, official daughter school to my alma mater in Johannesburg, leased a large and well-lit second-floor office space right off the town square.

Several of those serendipitous guests to our facility became my good friends - like Mark Saito, 10th-dan rising lineage holder of Shorinjin Ryu Ninjitsu. For a short while in the mid-1990s, we had a venture together to teach life skills based upon the inner principles of martial arts to teenagers at risk.The results were quite remarkable—until our state funding dried up. One of the class exercises seemed odd at first, but turned out to be especially valuable. Mark would have us go out into the woods, armed with our *shinai* (bamboo kendo practice sword). Each student would find a tree—which then became his or her sparring partner. A ready posture was adopted, and the students waited intently for their tree to let its guard down - at which point the tree would be swiftly attacked with a sword cut and a yell (*kiai*).

Never was a wood more silent. Because of course the trees never let down their guard. For every second of their long lives, they never stopped being a tree—not even for a moment. The trees stood as a perfect example of *zanshin*, a Japanese martial arts term meaning "restful alertness" (literally "remaining mind"). Wikipedia tells us that: "In the context of Kendo, *zanshin* is the continued state of mental alertness and physical readiness to instantly attack or respond to an attack or counter attack by one's opponent."

As soon as the mind wanders, we become identified with something outside of ourselves and zanshin is broken. It is so easy to see when someone's t'ai chi form becomes broken in this way. But this is only the beginning...

The two essential constituents of *zanshin* in martial arts are awareness and intention. Any physical conditioning, or combat techniques we learn, are meaningless outside of the context of these two foundational traits. From a simplistic standpoint, awareness is the basis of defense, and intention the basis of offense. A particular emphasis in t'ai chi is that our environment extends inwards to what's going on within our own body as much as it applies to the opponent and external surroundings. They're all part of a continuous (not contiguous) system. The exercises of Push Hands and *San Shou* (scattered hands, the two-man form) develop awareness and intention in the external continuum, whereas the basic t'ai chi form tends to develop awareness and intention internally.

The basis of *zanshin*, restful alertness, or awareness and intention, is Presence. The basis of effective living is Presence. Thus the martial arts are such a wonderful metaphor for life in general. In dealing totally pragmatically with the most stressful and horrific aspects of human interaction on the battlefield, they certainly also provide proven psycho-physiological strategies for dealing with the mundane.

We have seen that the t'ai chi *diagram* is about dynamism, about movement, about the mechanics of unmanifest Being becoming. In movement, the t'ai chi *form* outwardly expresses all the features of the invisible micro-scale processes of creation and evolution in the macro-scale world of our senses—if we have presence, awareness and intention.

The human body was designed to move. Many of our modern ills stem directly from our sedentary lifestyles. I understand the value of ch'i kung (*qigong*) and yoga exercises for firing the engines and clearing out channels and pathways. But although it's much more complex, t'ai chi provides all of those benefits, and more—because all aspects of the entire physiology are in motion. As a compromise, if you need to really stretch organs and tendons, plus get the energy moving, then t'ai chi's 800-year-old Taoist cousin, pa tuan chin (*baduanjin*—eight section brocade) will definitely help. Again I believe a primary reason for its remarkable effectiveness is that the performer is for the most part moving.

In my travels I have witnessed three major training philosophies in t'ai chi teachers:

i) those that emphasize building organic strength and rooting to support the required experience;

ii) those that focus on synchrony of breath and energy circuits; and

iii) those that pay special consideration to the quality of attention, leaving the internal technical detail to Nature.

Of course, all of these are important. However, my sifu subscribed to the third category (with a generous sum of the first included). The idea was that our bodies had innate intelligence and would spontaneously figure out what to do with energy and breathing if we just practiced the postures correctly—putting the body in a configuration conducive to the desired result—and put our undivided attention on what was going on inside.

I find now that I am comfortably across the boundary of my second half-century, I have lost a lot of my enthusiasm for "eating bitter". I still like to train hard, but only to the point where the experience remains sweet. The focus of my practice has become exploring spirituality and presence—and besides, my knees are quite militantly opposed to the exertions once expected of them. Whatever the reasons for our study, the approach to training should be the same. Whether one takes meditation for enlightenment or to relieve a headache, if the discipline is approached with the correct attitude, one will gain the best possible outcome.

So remain soft, pliant—stay present while paying attention to the Form surging and rippling through every joint and sinew. The classics say: the mind leads the ch'i (*qi*), and the ch'i leads the body. Intention, attention, and awareness.

My middle teens were spent growing up next to the river in a tiny rural village about 30 miles southeast of Johannesburg. Whereas most kids visit each other on bicycles, we tended to do it by canoe. The father of one of my friends a couple of miles downstream had patented a garden watering device he invented. It was completely ingenious in its simplicity. No moving parts—just a tripod stand perhaps five feet high, with a garden hose led up and attached to the top. There was another five feet or so of hose left loose through the top of the stand. When the water was turned on, the pressure caused the extra length of hose to thrash around powerfully—sending a stream of water randomly in all directions. It was fascinating to watch, this hose with a haunting life of its own as a result of the water flowing through it.

The novel garden sprinkler gave me an idea for a most valuable exercise in our t'ai chi classes—the seaweed exercise. My students really didn't care for it in the beginning because it made them feel very self-conscious. But I liked it, so we did it anyway. It was an exercise in awareness, intention and attention—but presence and self-consciousness don't fit together very well, so it was a good exercise from that point of view too. Students had to pretend that they were seaweed growing viably in the ocean. From their knees down, they imagined that they were anchored into the bed of the sea. Their hips and waist were the seaweed's trunk, and their hands, arms and shoulders were the seaweed fronds in the water current. If they lost their root (feet, ankles and knees became brittle and disconnected), then they would find themselves washed up on the sun-bleached beaches of Australia—a fate worse than death. If their trunk snapped (hips weren't open, or waist failed to twist flexibly and transfer the energy from the root), then they would be washed away and wind up on the sun-bleached beaches of Australia—a fate worse than death. If their flowing fronds became stiff and broke in the current (the arms lost their pliancy and failed to follow the direction from the waist), then they would find themselves washed up on the sun-bleached beaches of Australia…

When the exercise was properly executed, our movements were graceful, fluid and very much like Arthur Waldron's gyrating garden sprinkler. Instead of worrying what we looked like (faintly absurd), we paid attention to what we felt inside. When the desire to move (our idea of the sea current) arose within the *dan tien* and waist, it was manifested in the arms and upper body like the water pressure animating the hose. And by remaining aware of our lively connection to the ground, we were able to project that intention of movement out into the fingertips. It felt good. The field of dreams materialized. Was this heaven? No it was Iowa. And we had escaped dry oblivion on the shores of Australia…

You can not do the seaweed exercise credibly without folding. This means that the end of one motion is folded into the beginning of the next.

The mind moves the ch'i, and the ch'i moves the body. Baby Boomer readers may have watched the earlier days of television mentioned in the introduction. If so, you may remember the phenomenon of red flare. This was an artifact of differing response times for the light sensing elements of the old Plumbicon television camera tube. If you watched, say, a trumpeter and the stage lights were reflecting off his instrument, then as he moved, there would be a swath of red following the gleaming movement of the trumpet. This effect was produced because the red signal in the studio camera lagged behind the rest of the spectrum. Just like that, the outward movement of the body is like the red image—although absolutely connected, it follows a little way behind the real picture, which is the intention encoded in the flowing ch'i.

The mind moves the ch'i, and the ch'i moves the body. And the quiet Self present in the *dan tien* witnesses it all without becoming involved. In order to experience how different qualities of awareness express themselves in our Form and to firmly establish the Form as a conscious expression of our awareness, we would sometimes put the mind in an unfamiliar framework. We'd do silly things, like pretending to do the routine on Jupiter where we were immensely heavier than was our normal experience in Iowa—making it harder to express the sprouting ch'i through dense, cumbersome limbs. Or on Mercury, where we were so light, it was difficult to maintain a solid root and control fly-away extremities.

The least attractive part about our club's training area in Fairfield was the carpet. A sprung wood floor would have been nice, but membership fees were minimal and all the room boasted was an old industrial fitted carpet. It was a kind of nondescript, grayish brindle burlap, made up of small blotches of black, light grey and brown. How could that most unprepossessing feature of the school be turned to our advantage?

If you imagined yourself to be an enormous giant, then those flecks and blotches in the carpet looked like little villages and a patchwork of fields way down below. You were a mighty god, the lord of all you surveyed. As you moved through the Form, entire populations lived or got squished at your pleasure. Would you defend your people against other marauding giants—or wreak havoc in their world? It was very interesting to do the Form with this sense of omnipotence and compassion. The innocent result was great silence—a class full of inwardly directed and very mindful people performing research into the mechanics of consciousness. To the observer, they all looked very regal—a room full of kings and queens practicing a very powerful and expansive Form (with some impressive control displayed in footwork).

Enough with the stories. We have discussed how, through the "eyes", the fully expressed value of *yang* collapses onto its point value—which is *yin*. And that fully retracted *yin* implodes into the outward expression of *yang* again. We saw how the *yin* collapse in the lower *dan tien* produces lively *jing* (***agni***), and that *yang* collapse in the head centers creates the ***soma*** condensate. This is the natural rhythm of things, but it can be augmented and amplified by conscious attention and intention. These motivators are under the direction of the middle *dan tien*, the energy field of the heart, which is the seat of intention.

This process is reflected in the t'ai chi Form. When a movement or posture reaches its culmination (ward-off, for example), then its quality collapses into its antithesis and the movement and direction are reversed. The full becomes empty. In roll-back, the *yin* collapses into young *yang* and the empty returns to full. And so on. When we are present, we can delve consciously and deeply into the mechanics of the collapse. The collapse presents outwardly as folding and plaiting. For the casual observer, it isn't possible to see where one movement ends and the next begins. There must be a terminus, but the entire body responds like a segmented spring—so it's fluid and the collapse happens in a whip-like sequence.

Practicing the t'ai chi form is like being a researcher in a living laboratory. We take the theory and scientific drawings from the t'ai chi diagram and give them tangible expression. The mind moves the ch'i, and the ch'i moves the body. And the quiet Self present in the *dan tien* witnesses it all without becoming involved. There is transcendence, there is fixity of attention, and there is the movement of intention—all together.

And the kicker? Who says the collapse, the transformation, has to happen at the fullest (Ch'ien and K'un) points in the cycle? This is how we take a science and make it a technology. This is the relationship of t'ai chi to the Tao. Before we move onto an analysis of how we can consciously manage and direct the process of transformation and creation, I want to introduce one last iteration of the diagram that emphasizes the cardinal points. These four areas (Chien, Li, K'an and K'un) are the seats of prime influence.

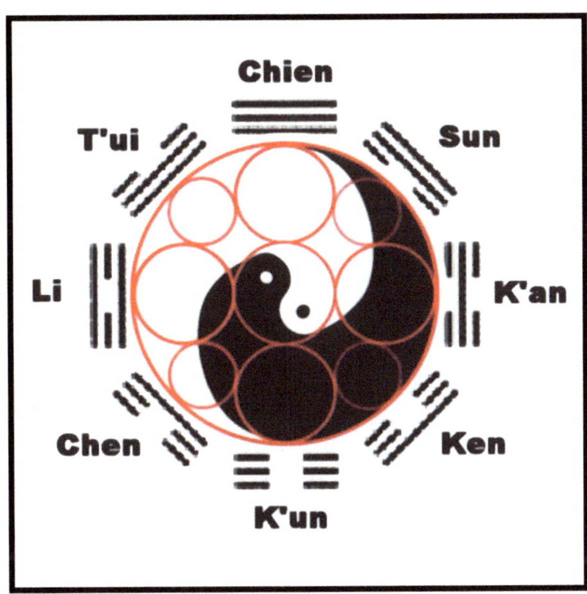

七

SAMYAMA

It isn't my purpose to discuss the details of actual t'ai chi forms, nor to offer any recommendations for classical correct practice such as Yang Cheng-fu's famous 10 main points, for instance. Rather, this is a deliberation of the consciousness aspects of the practice—a sort of meta-t'ai chi.

If you're folding properly while practicing your t'ai chi form, you will experience heat in the palms or fingers during the fold as the ch'i exudes, streams, or spurts forth from the collapse. The timing of the transition into the next posture in the sequence is determined by the quality of the emission. Sending out energy in this way is very much like throwing out a toy yo-yo. There is a rhythm involved. And until the yo-yo returns to your hand, you are exposed and vulnerable.

In similar fashion to the fact that the earth's path around the sun represents its shortest, most efficient path through the cosmos, I also believe that in the e-space of our

Form, the quality of the fold demonstrates our progress toward the path of greatest efficiency. It is the path through our environment that creates least disturbance.

My nervous system is not given to bling or flashy experiences, so I don't get to see auras in sparkling technicolor. Nevertheless, I do sense energy fields as a sort of filmy substance, and it gave me the idea for one other "game" that we used to sometimes play with the Form. It was called the Will-O'-the-Wisp form. A will-o'-the-wisp is a fleeting ethereal spirit that drifts through the swirling mists and vapors that hang and sprawl over the English moors. The objective of this form was to cause as little disruption in the surrounding mist as possible. In a clumsy execution, one could visualize the full extension at the end of a movement as causing a swirling vortex in the mist. If you folded carefully, you could cut a path through the mist that didn't create wild eddies that spun off from your transitions.

Of course, there are instances where we want to create powerful waves at points of our choosing (*fajing*). This is the subject of this chapter.

The t'ai chi classics describe correct performance as being like threading pearls on a necklace. Each posture (Single-Whip, White Crane Spreads Wings, etc.) is like a pearl. But the Form only arises by the smooth connection likened to the threading of the pearls into a string. So what's more important? The pearls that you see, or the threads that you don't?

We will look at this by investigating the ancient Vedic prescriptions for engineering the process of manifestation. The information is encapsulated as aphorisms, called ***sutras*** in Sanskrit—which literally means "threads".

In the Bhagavad Gita, that great distillation of the essence of Vedic wisdom, we read: ***"Nistraigunyo bhav, Arjuna*** (Be without the three ***gunas***, Arjuna – II.45)." And then

"Yogastha kuru karmani (Established in Being, perform action—II.48)." The sequence is important here and applies directly to the practice of t'ai chi ch'uan. Lord Krishna admonishes Arjuna to leave behind the field of multiplicity, to transcend and experience Unity. By getting our awareness out of the field of day-to-day relative concerns, the field of the Three, we return to the One. Once our awareness is established in pure consciousness, then only can we be assured of performing effective and appropriate action. To rephrase, the instruction is: "Transcend and *then* Act." The basis of successful action in the field of the Three is to have our awareness permanently infused with the One.

The beginning of the Form is of profound importance. I always think to myself: "If I could just get the opening sequence down. The rest would just be frosting on the cake…"

Any solo empty-handed t'ai chi form that I remember learning, whatever the style, had an opening sequence where the practitioner stepped out into a horse stance to begin. The start of the Yang Form, and the official Simplified Taiji derivative, has us standing with the feet together. When it's time to begin, we are taught to empty our minds of extraneous outside thoughts. We step out with our feet a shoulder-width apart and commence with raising the arms, extending the fingers and then withdrawing back down before turning for Ward-Off Left (or Parting the Wild Horse's Mane).

As a novice, I remember being very impatient with Sifu Eddie. What was taking so long? Why couldn't we get going with the Raise Hands already? After we had stepped into the parallel stance, it seemed like forever before we got started.

If you think that the Form begins with Raise Hands, you've already missed it. The outward Form is really just a commentary on what has already happened—very like our earlier analysis of "Rig Veda" as the commentary of its very first syllable.

As we step across to start the Form, our awareness centers and condenses. It drains away from the edges and congeals. Once resolved, it drops like a stone into the *dan tien* as the left foot steps down and makes root. And then it's almost as though the Form emerges from the splash.

Without first establishing presence, the awareness cannot be gathered. We lose the basis for this resolution of consciousness that collapses to give birth to all the subsequent expressions of the Form. The quality of the practice is determined by the clarity of this initial experience immediately before the outward form begins.

The first four sutras of chapter three of Patanjali's "Yoga Sutras" describe what constitutes the practice of ***samyama*** (pronounced more like sanyama).

> i) ***Dharana*** or attention is the mind's fixation on a particular point in space.
>
> ii) In that attention, the continuous flow of the same knowledge is called ***Dhyana***.
>
> iii) When the distinctions between object and subject are eliminated, and our true nature alone shines forth in the mind, then this is called ***Samadhi***.
>
> iv) The three together simultaneously is called ***Samyama***.

In other words, if you have fixation, movement, and transcendence—all at once—then you have ***samyama***. This at first sounds like a completely self-contradictory collection of requirements and through the centuries there has been much misunderstanding regarding the procedure. However, there are clearly defined techniques to achieve ***samyama***—and I believe that t'ai chi ch'uan can be one of them.

In the "Yoga Sutras", Patanjali provides specific formulas of ***samyama*** practice to produce desired effects in consciousness that create corresponding results in the gross physical realm—special powers such as supernormal hearing, increased compassion, or levitation. Such supernormal abilities are traditionally called ***siddhis***. ***Samyama*** is the method for directly acting within the Gap, the technique for initiating action right in the boundary zone between absolute (the One) and relative (the Three). At this level of the t'ai chi diagram, one can determine the outcome of the collapse—we specify what qualities are to be brought forth out of the Gap, the fully customized collapse of the wave function in the quantum field.

I have watched hundreds of new initiates' bodily reactions to the internal release of energy through their spinal columns when they begin to experience ***samyama*** in sitting meditation. But I have also watched the release of energy in students learning Grandmaster Hsiung's T'ai Chi Dao Yin. And I have seen even more students' convulsive signs of their first elementary experiences of *fa jing*. To my eyes, in all cases the more refined nervous systems spontaneously had exactly the same symptoms.

If you ponder Patanjali's stipulations, you realize that ***samyama*** is precisely what correct t'ai chi form exercises and requires. It must be noted that the majority of my t'ai chi students were long-term practitioners of the Transcendental Meditation (TM) and TM-Sidhi techniques—and so came to the Form with a solid understanding of the principles, plus extensive experience in two of the indispensable elements, viz. transcendence (***Samadhi***) and meditation (***Dhyan***). In this sense, I was afforded a head start in researching this aspect of t'ai chi. The Form was a wonderful outlet and application for their skills, and they progressed very quickly once the basic postures and sequence of movements of the Form were learned. On the other hand, their t'ai chi practice also became a powerful opportunity for growing in and integrating higher levels of consciousness.

With all martial arts, the forms and techniques are practiced over and over until they become a reflexive organic memory in our muscles and nervous systems. We don't have to think *how* to do the movements on the outside anymore, we're free to focus on the refinement of *what* to do inside.

So we practice diligently, until the Form is an unconsciously integral part of us. After that, it's not so much us doing the Form, as the Form doing us. But still we pay minute attention as it unfolds. With all our intention, we still lead the ch'i onward to unveil each move as though it were the first time. And all the while there is that settled awareness, the silent witness centered in the lower *dan tien*.

Again, the most marvelous thing about the t'ai chi form is that while all this stuff is going on internally, it is also reflected in movement externally. In this way, every level of our being is involved and exercised in the practice.

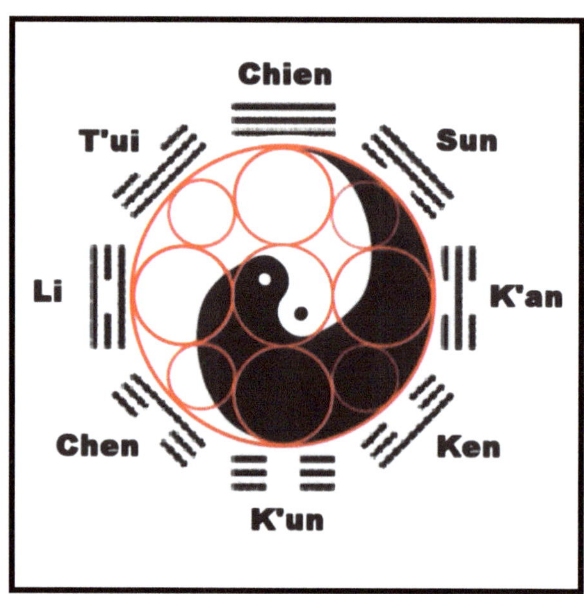

During regular repetition of the Form, each movement swells to its point of maximum expression and then folds into the start of the following posture. Full becomes empty, empty becomes full. And so the pearls are threaded together.

The natural cycle has the *yang* collapse at the Chien point (e.g. ward-off), and the yin collapse at the K'un point (e.g. roll-back). But these are not the optimal points to either release an attack, or to absorb or deflect an attack from your opponent. These places of full extension are vulnerable with no room to maneuver.

At the Li point in the cycle, *yang* is expressed in the subject (heaven) and object (earth) positions, but there is a *yin* line in the motivating process (man) position. Intention will cause the collapse of the *yin* into *yang*, making the full power of Chien explosively available at the most favorable part of the movement's evolution. Often this gives rise to a characteristic, almost involuntary double contraction. There is risk here because Chien is unstable. If the *fa jing* is defeated, then the emitter is exposed (like the released yo-yo) until the ch'i returns for a further collapse into the *yin* stage, and so on.

Likewise, the K'an point is the most sensitive scenario in the withdrawal phase. Through conscious intention, the collapse of the *yang* line in the dynamism place of the trigram results in the completely *yin* status of K'un. The attack will be smothered and neutralized, and the attacker's energy returned circularly as the empty implodes back into a *yang* mode.

As such, the Li and K'an positions have the greatest potential for manifesting change. This is a deeper level of ***samyama*** practice in the Form. As I have observed, these events happen spontaneously with the development of our practice. The really exciting part is being aware of what's happening and growing to be aware of each nuance of the process.

This is how the magic comes through training. At the school, we were once given a seminar by a visiting world champion t'ai chi player. He is the rising head of a very venerable family in the Yang-style tradition. But he told us that in his opinion there was no such thing as magic in t'ai chi. He considered *fa li* (issuing strength) and *fa jing* (emitting energy) to be synonymous. The martial arts are a very practical subject. On the ground, you can either deliver the goods, or you can't. So it's hard to argue with the world champion. But I saw a video of his grandfather demonstrating the Form—and there was magic if ever I saw it.

In the same way that a tree is always a tree, and a dog is always a dog (how do they learn to know us so well?), the best way to progress as a student is to empty your cup, be your natural uncomplicated self, and pay meticulous attention to the teacher. In my early days with Sifu Eddie Jardine, I managed this to some measure. Courtesy was paramount, but Eddie wasn't one for standing on ceremony and always expressed a cordial dislike for organized showmanship. Nonetheless, there was always perfect discipline at the school. People trained at his dojo because of what he was, and if he chose (as he usually did, and we wouldn't have dreamt of doing) to train barefoot in a t-shirt and shorts, then everyone willingly accorded him a much higher level of respect than many less capable yet crisply uniformed tyrants—whatever their rank and self-assumed importance.

Apart from his internationally recognized mastery, Eddie is an immensely strong man. You didn't want him to get a hold of you. And he didn't appear to feel the cold either. So it was with some surprise and concern that at one point I noticed that he had been instructing for some time in a sweatsuit, socks and sneakers. I asked him about it and he spoke as though very reluctant to accept what he was saying. A while earlier, Eddie's teacher, Duan Sifu had returned to Taiwan from a visit to us in South Africa. Before he left, apparently he had simply touched Eddie's arm. Eddie had felt some weakness and been told that Sifu had taken his *yang* energy. Not to worry, he had been assured, after a few weeks it would return. Eddie couldn't understand it. He said he felt cold through to his bones, and had felt that way for weeks. No such thing as magic? Duan Sifu specialized in such demonstrations. This story is one of the less phenomenal.

Our visiting push-hands champion was right. There is no such thing as magic. It's just an unusual facility in working in the Gap. But that's very different from a physical mastery of applied mechanics or *fa li*. In the next chapter we'll look at how these inner technologies express themselves in everyday life.

OUTSIDE THE PRACTICE

Unless you're an audiophile with a lot of time and money, it is probably easier and safer to purchase a home theater system from a single reputable vendor. In that way you know that the sound and video will be of high quality and all the components will hook together easily and without any incompatibilities.

As far as a system for the theater of real life is concerned, the t'ai chi diagram and its Taoist underpinnings is a one-stop solution also. It is very satisfying that the philosophy (as encapsulated in the diagram) for the evolution of the cosmos, at the same time, provides the framework for the system of martial arts—which is also the best form of general wellness training, plus the basis of prophylactic measures against aging, and ties precisely into the traditional system of medicine… And can be used to manage our day to day business of living. The whole system is self-referral and one hundred percent internally congruent. In previous chapters, we took recourse to the Vedic texts of ancient India. But that was to explain and illuminate, not because of any insufficiency in the t'ai chi perspective.

Looking outside the practice of t'ai chi ch'uan we find two directions: one more outward in the expressed values of everyday life, and the other quieter and more introspective.

Let's turn to look at the inner basis of the practice first, because enriching that area of our lives adds great value to both the t'ai chi form and outer life.

I had mentioned that the majority of my t'ai chi students were advanced meditators and skilled at working with the group dynamics of consciousness. Although this is not essential for becoming proficient in the t'ai chi form, and one can get by in life without it, in order to enjoy ever more refined levels of experience and intuitively grasp deeper values of the t'ai chi diagram, a program of internal practice is definitely recommended.

Unfortunately, over the course of thirty years I have only ever met one t'ai chi specialist who I considered to be both competent and willing to offer any training in productive meditation. So that's a bit limiting from a t'ai chi perspective if you want to remain in the one-stop shopping paradigm. As a teacher of Transcendental Meditation since the tail-end of the 1970s, I can vouch for the enormous benefits that accrue from that simple and scientifically validated mediation practice (www.TM.org). However, many people don't want to mix their cultural traditions, or are nervous about getting involved with anything they might associate (rightly or wrongly) with a particular belief system. For those "show me" t'ai chi players who are looking to increase their level of awareness and sensitivity, but want a simple method with absolutely no philosophical connections or connotations, I heartily recommend Holosync brainwave entrainment technology from the Centerpointe Research Institute (www.centerpointe.com).

Obviously the next stage outward from the t'ai chi form involves the art in conjunction with other people—starting with the Push Hands techniques and Two-Man form.

Probably the most well-known exponent of the Two-Man form (t'ai chi san shou) in the United States was the late T. T. Liang. Like Master Liang, I was fortunate to have learned the form from the great Taiwanese legend, Grandmaster Hsiung (*Xiong*). Early one morning I was going through the san shou form with *sigong* when I had perhaps one of the weirdest "twilight zone" experiences of my life. Following the set sequence, I had punched and Master Hsiung had executed the appropriate block. My punch was stopped and my arm trapped in the specified way. I couldn't move, and I could see his fingers stretched around my wrist and forearm. But for a second I just stared at my wrist nonplussed—because I couldn't *feel* his grasp. He held me fast, but he was so in tune with my energy that I couldn't feel it at all. Somewhat shaken, I turned to face him again, and he was looking straight into my eyes with that inscrutable little Chinese smile.

I loved Master Hsiung very much. You couldn't help it. He emanated a sort of warm settled glow that felt like coming home. Accomplished martial arts masters tend to be gifted healers. It comes with the territory. I have known several great champions who practiced their art because they loved it, and healed because they were called to it—and because attending to people's ills paid the bills better. But Hsiung Wei didn't have to touch you. You simply felt better by being around him.

The most immediately noticeable thing to spill out of the practice of t'ai chi and into the regular world is the quality of breath. Back when I was starting, I don't remember Duan Sifu ever asking us to control the rhythm of the breath during the Form —we were asked to breath naturally. But in any martial art, breathing needs to be diaphragmatic in order to sink and control the energy. To help with this, we were taught to imagine that we had a tube or straw coming out of our navels while training and to breathe through that—a most effective visualization. Once established in the body as an unconscious habit, this style of abdominal breathing—that more closely mirrors the cycles of the t'ai chi diagram—is of inestimable value. It directly impacts every area of our general health, and also our ability to approach life from the settled perspective of the One.

In our world of ubiquitous personal computers there are new fun ways to test and further exercise the energy and breath control that spontaneously develops through t'ai chi. The Journey to Wild Divine (www.wilddivine.com) is an interactive computer game that requires a high degree of command over breath, heart rate, stress response, and so on.

In the coming sections we will look at how the t'ai chi diagram is just as effective in organizing and explaining our outer environment as it is in describing the rudiments and expression of the t'ai chi form. We will see the value of training ourselves to locate the One in the midst of the Three (and all of diversity) whatever our field of endeavor.

The traditional oriental strategy game of *Go* emphasizes the concept of having *sente*—which means "having the initiative". Without *sente*, you cannot control your destiny—your every move is simply a defensive response to those of your opponent. Similarly, in the martial arts and life as a whole, we are doomed unless we can determine and lead the rhythm with which events in our environment unfold.

In any enterprise, keeping *sente* involves maintaining a settled composure and a broad view of the circumstances, while at the same time being able to focus very sharply on details at hand. Psychologists call this field independence—the ability to concentrate on particulars without losing the perspective of the whole. It's really just an application of maintaining the One and the Three simultaneously. Strength in the field of the Three is augmented and supported by the quality of our conscious infusion of the One. This is what the t'ai chi diagram tells us—always Three *and* One—and further that by acting within the Gap, we can proactively influence events for the best outcome for ourselves and our environment. This is sometimes called gaining the "support of Nature."

Continuously evident field independence and pronounced creativity both require a high level of coherence in brain functioning. Increased brainwave coherence means greater orderliness in the nervous system—which in turn correlates with higher levels of consciousness. Life experiences in general, and internal martial arts in particular, are a clear and empirical test of our achievements in developing higher states of consciousness.

The natural tendency of the inanimate universe is to degenerate towards a more entropic or disorderly condition. In contrast, the prime characteristic of living systems is that they can maintain a high degree of ordered structure over extended periods of time. By extracting order and energy from the surroundings, all living organisms manage to go against the basic inclination of their chaotic environment and persist at a thermodynamic distance from it. In addition, the self-referral, self-repairing nature of DNA, the blueprint of life, allows for life to be perpetuated across generations indefinitely. More evolved creatures display a proportionately greater degree of order and differentiation in their structure, metabolism, and emotional and mental capacity.

As members of the human race, we have been endowed with astonishing physical, mental, and spiritual faculties. However, in order to accommodate and express the perfect orderliness of the Gap, in order to be able to permanently hold in our awareness the One together with the Three, the nervous system has to evolve. It has to be restructured in greater complexity, exercised and integrated.

In the context of t'ai chi, it is said that we learn the teacher, not the Form. There is a level of organic body-mind learning that occurs completely below our conscious awareness. Many have noted that the experience of practicing t'ai chi in a group is very different from solo performance. Being in a group greatly facilitates this subliminal learning effect—and there is a powerful reason for it.

Even a small fraction of individuals behaving coherently within a group facilitates a phase transition to greater orderliness within the entire group. This is a well understood principle of physics called super-radiance, and describes the basis of light stimulation in a laser. Just the square root of one percent of atoms in the laser emitting light coherently excites all the others to do the same. This light source, where all emitted photons have exactly the same wavelength and propagate in phase, results in a beam many thousands of times more powerful than an incandescent light of the same power consumption. The whole is much greater than the sum of its parts.

And consciousness follows the same pattern. The first time I set foot in the United States was during the winter holidays of 1983. It was a shock—coming from a beautiful South African midsummer to the middle of a record-setting Iowa winter with reported wind chills of –60 degrees Fahrenheit. I arrived in Fairfield with a group of South Africans to participate in the greatest experiment and demonstration of the group dynamics of consciousness that the world has ever seen. At that time, the square root of one percent of the world's population was about 7,000. We managed to assemble almost 8,000 pioneers to practice TM and ***samyama***, diving into the Gap together. The effects measured included a reduction in world conflict and accident rates, and conversely increases in patent applications and positive stock market movements. The statistics were highly significant and all the more impressive because we predicted them in advance.

After that historic assembly, I remained in Fairfield until early 1984 to attend a leadership conference. It was there at Maharishi University of Management (then called Maharishi International University) that I remember first learning to build Unified Field Charts.

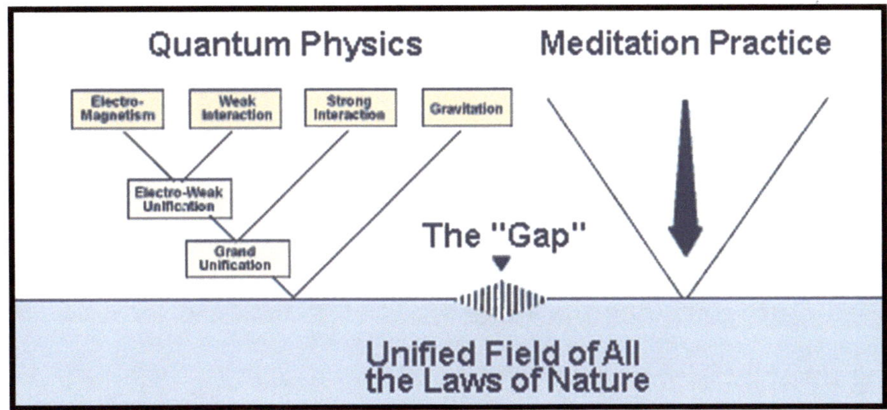

Unified Field Charts were invented by Maharishi to help enliven the connection between the One (unity) and the Three (diversity) in every area of organization. The chart has two parallel components:

i) on the right side is shown how the mind settles into the field of pure consciousness through meditation; and

ii) the left side of the diagram shows the progressive differentiation of the field of interest from the unified field of the all the laws of nature (vacuum state of the quantum field), through to the most surface level of the matter under review. Pure

Consciousness (ultimate subjective reality) and the Vacuum State of the Quantum Field (ultimate objective reality) are considered to be synonymous.

So, for example, the Unified Field Chart for the human physiology (a chart for a health professional) might show the following levels from finest to most expressed:

i) the level of the Unified Field;

ii) Bose and Fermi fields giving rise to the four fundamental forces of physics (weak, strong, electromagnetic, gravitational), plus quarks, leptons and neutrinos (representing the matter fields);

iii) differentiating further to give rise to atoms and molecules, the building blocks of DNA;

iv) expressed as proteins;

v) giving structure to cell components;

vi) making up cells;

vii) constituting tissues;

vii) comprising organs;

viii) combining to form systems;

ix) resulting in the individual physiology; and

x) and from there through society right up to the group physiology of national government.

I have always found the charts very constructive in channeling my attention on the inner values of any situation or enterprise—and they prompted me to do the same thing with the t'ai chi diagram. In a sense, it is a unified field chart also, but with a slightly different perspective. It looks at a surface circumstance and relates it directly to the fundamentals of the One (***samhita***/wu chi), the Three (knower, known and process of knowing), and the 8 essential natures of the bagua.

This methodology can be applied to any group or community—such as families, clubs, institutions of learning, or government. However, these collections of individuals do not have an independent existence of their own. They are intended to exist only to provide a framework for the activities of their members. As such they are really a natural outgrowth of our social disposition. There is another kind of entity that warrants closer attention.

Perhaps the most surprising and often disturbing aspect of our current civilization is the megalithic corporation. There is intense scientific research and all kinds of ethical furor over the creation of artificial life. But of course, Frankenstein in the guise of a corporation began to take shape several hundred years ago. Corporations fulfill every defining characteristic of a living organism that I can think of. In the modern world, corporations as living entities have all the legal and social rights, and none of the physical frailties, of their creators. Employees are the equivalent of cells, departments are like organs, and we even talk about the "body corporate".

Of course, being the creation of man and not the product of Nature, corporations have been built using only partial access to the field of all the laws of Nature. Being solely a reflection of the Three, they were not fashioned in accord with the t'ai chi diagram that takes into account the One—which contains within it all the laws of Nature in their seed form. Thus a fragmented basis gives rise to results that don't express the full value of the force of cosmic evolution. Without lively recourse to the unified field of the One, a corporation's self-serving interests cannot provide a life-supporting influence for all. As such, corporations suffer from the same shortcomings and conflicts that plague individuals trapped in a totally materialistic world view. Because their plans and actions are not based in pure awareness, their goals tend to be short-sighted, and they suffer internally and are the subject of malicious competition in the marketplace. In the end they threaten to usurp the freedoms, and compete brutally for the wealth and resources of their biological counterparts.

In this way, corporations are like surrogates for our own foibles, and the economics of the corporate world very much resembles a battlefield amongst peoples.

Almost all of us expend most of our life's energy in some form of company environment, so it would be useful to see how the t'ai chi diagram, and the principles of the martial arts, can be applied to the corporate world. Not in the Sun Tzu ("The Art of War") sense of subterfuge and manipulation, but in the same vein as we have studied the t'ai chi material to elucidate and deepen our experience of the Form. The analysis of organizational dynamics is a whole new universe of application of the t'ai chi diagram.

Instead of looking out towards the Three from within the One—which has been our approach so far—an examination of the corporate environment seeks to rediscover the One from the churning commotion of the Three. Discovering how the t'ai chi diagram illuminates the dynamics of the workplace is of particular interest to business managers and anyone interested in developing a more evolved workplace.

Because the methodology for analyzing and evaluating organizational structure is reiterative and can drill into any level of managerial detail, and the model is self-referral in nature, I call it "**Recursive Organizational Dynamics**" (or ROD). Spare the ROD and ruin the company. As this area of investigation is quite complex and highly specialized, this will be the subject of a separate volume.

For now, it's enough to know that the fascinating new arena of Recursive Organizational Dynamics can be used to map both the obvious and hidden relationships, as well as the mutual interactions that make up the ongoing workings of any organization. A detailed ROD analysis of a modern company or department can be used to show the Gap transformations of Lao Tzu (as illuminated throughout this book by Vedic Science), bringing ancient and modern methodologies into perfect harmony.

Going beyond the basic characterization of the relationships between the various *bagua*, to fully analyze any situation in the outside world, requires looking at how events dynamically change and evolve. This can be achieved through studying the collapse of individual lines in their corresponding *bagua* trigrams—which explains the mechanics of evolution of any given circumstance. It is possible to actually see the patterns and blueprints of interaction between the *bagua* as they are unwaveringly structured by the permutations permitted by the intrinsic nature of the Gap (as expressed by the t'ai chi diagram). The only certainty about relative existence is change. Understanding change is what the t'ai chi diagram is about. Managing change is what trigram line changes and the "eyes" of the diagram are about—the process of engineering reality through the mechanics of the Gap.

The trigrams were originally conceived almost 5,000 years ago. Then about 1,150 BCE in the early Chou dynasty, King Wen, original author of the venerable I-Ching, devised a way to enumerate and explain the relationships between the eight basic natural tendencies (or *bagua*) that the trigrams represent. He did this by looking at the qualities expressed by viewing each trigram in relation to each other trigram. These relationships are drawn by stacking the subject and object trigrams over each other, yielding a 6-lined glyph called a hexagram. There are therefore 64 hexagrams and these make up the subject matter of the I-Ching. King Wen ascribed certain attributes to each hexagram that characterized the relationship it depicted. He gave each hexagram a name and summary, plus some advice for dealing with the situation. It is said that the I-Ching has a definite personality. Working with the I-Ching requires practice and familiarity, but the effort is rewarding. After a while, it seems as though we're listening to a wise old sage talking through the symbolism of the hexagrams. And of course, that wise old sage is Nature, because the I-Ching and the t'ai chi diagram are both simply tools to magnify, illuminate and explain the intrinsic fabric of creation.

The hexagrams and the various commentaries of the I-Ching offer a succinct description of overall functional relationships between the eight *bagua* trigrams, but we have not addressed Gap transformations. Remember that a transformation occurs when a yin or yang line reaches its extremity, becomes unstable, and collapses through the Gap into its opposite. The I-Ching specifically involves the mapping of Gap transformations. These changing elements are called "moving lines" in the text. When a component line in a hexagram mutates into its complement, then the first hexagram transforms into another because of the line change.

Thousands of years ago, King Wen's son, the Duke of Chou, added the analysis of what it meant if any constituent line in a hexagram changed. History's greatest scholar of the I-Ching was perhaps Confucius (551-479 BCE)—who edited the material and provided additional commentaries and annotations to form the text that is available to us today. So it is a book of great antiquity. Through hexagram symbolism and tracking line changes, the I-Ching, the millennia-old Chinese book of divination, predicts the evolution of events in the phenomenal world. We can use it to understand processes as they happen.

Following the unfoldment of situations through line changes is very precise, but can get quite complicated. ROD diagrams place the changes in a structured framework that makes patterns easier to spot and reveals the underlying mechanics of evolution. Whatever your work or sphere of influence, going through the exercise of building these charts for your own situation will certainly be instructive—if not revelatory.

Since this I-Ching-oriented analysis takes into account the fundamental patterns of manifestation from out of the Gap, it serves to make clear the imperceptible energetic basis for the functioning and relationships between the participants within any group. We are afforded a glimpse into the workings of Nature and the underlying mechanics of unfoldment in any given situation. Seen in this unusual light, many novel strategies present themselves for managing the development and deployment of an effective operational framework. It will be fundamentally instructive to elucidate these underlying associations as a basis for performance measurement and personnel management.

Readers who are already familiar with the I-Ching have perhaps had an uneasiness lingering in the back of their minds since the early "3-in-1" chapter. When comparing the structure and evolution of the trigrams and hexagrams in relation to the unfoldment of creation according to Rig Veda, we noted that Rig Veda espoused 192 modalities of manifestation. In review, there were 8 basic natures (or ***prakritis***) that were analyzed in terms of knower, process and known (***rishi, devata*** and ***chhandas***). Each of those 24 was then seen in relation to each of the 8 ***prakritis*** to yield a total of 192 ***suktas*** (or verses). By simple associative arithmetic, we restated this as 64 permutations of nature viewed by 3 vantages (knower, known and process). But the I-Ching deals with 384 mutations—because each of the 6 lines in each of the 64 hexagrams can transmute into its *yin/yang* counterpart. Thus the I-Ching deals with double the number of possibilities that are considered in the Rig Veda. In practice, there can be more than one line changing at any one time, allowing for a total or 4,096 permutations described by the I-Ching.

Nonetheless, there is no contradiction here. The I-Ching, as a system of divination, tracks any possible change in a particular circumstance. And any configuration of Natural Law can mutate into any other. Thus there are indeed 384 permutations. On the other hand, the Rig Veda seeks to describe relationships that give rise to specific configurations of consciousness. In this sense, the lower trigram represents the subject of a relationship, and the upper trigram is the quality related to. Only the subject trigram can reflect upon the different aspects of its configuration. Mutations in the upper trigram don't make any sense. So when looking at creative manifestation (as opposed to predictive analysis), only 192 permutations are allowed—giving rise to 512 possibilities when considering multiple simultaneous line changes. Each and all of the six lines in any hexagram can transmute into its complement. Any *yang* line can collapse in the Gap into a *yin* line, and vice versa. Changing lines cause a hexagram to transform into another hexagram, activating another part of the diagram.

Each group in society—whether it's a town, a country, a corporation, or football team—is made up of individuals. So far we've seen how the t'ai chi diagram makes clear the core mechanisms of creation and transformation from the point of view of the quietness of individual consciousness, to the gentle, measured practice of the t'ai chi form, and then the bustling chaos of the corporate world.

Let's go on to explore the societal ramifications of individuals infusing their awareness with the unchanging unified level of life.

九

1-IN-3

With the help of the t'ai chi diagram, we previously considered life force energy in terms of *yin* and *yang*, and in terms of the bodily expressions of the 3 fundamental aspects of reality - observer, observed and process. We also emphasized that the Three arise from the One, and that the story of the t'ai chi diagram is a commentary on the unfoldment of the Three from out of the One. While the One remains uninvolved, absolute and eternally non-changing, it is the source and goal of the ever-changing dynamism of the Three. The Three and their progressively more differentiated states constitute the domain of relativity. And the Gap is the lively interface between the One and the Three.

The essential structure of reality is expressed the same at any magnitude—emerging from the Gap at the Planck scale, to the microscopic, to the macroscopic, to the universal. Moreover, although we can harness the energies of ever finer strata of existence, the only possible way to effect change that is in accord with all the laws of Nature is to employ a technology that acts directly at the level of the Gap. When we delve beyond the finest strata of relativity, into the realm of the Gap, we pass into the field of pure subjectivity. To transcend means "to go beyond" and the Gap is the lively, dynamic quality of the Transcendent in the gap between the One and the Three. Emerging from here, the building blocks of the tangible world we know appear more like ideas than physical substance. The process of coalescence and sequential unfoldment of matter is a statistical summing of tendencies and possibilities, leading only to probabilities. If harnessed at this level, our desires and intentions have an immediate and unequivocal influence on the outcome of random fluctuations of the underlying Unified Field.

But by definition, any technology of the Gap (such as ***samyama*** or t'ai chi) must be a technology of consciousness. Beyond space, time and causation, the One cannot be probed objectively. It can only be experienced, researched, and known subjectively. The only machinery in the known universe for consciously exploring the absolute field of the One is the human nervous system. This is our greatest gift, and to waste it, or spend a life without even knowing it, is an unthinkable shame. T'ai chi is a wonderful exercise for integrating higher states of consciousness into the physiology—making ever more subtle modes of functioning a permanent reality of our day-to-day lives. However, the Form does not expand the container of consciousness. This was the point of Maharishi's cautionary comment—mentioned in the introduction to this book. The practice of t'ai chi is about moving ch'i through the body, and the fundamental axiom of the art points to the thing most needed: the mind moves the ch'i, and the ch'i moves the body. The mind comes first. There has to be some discipline for developing awareness if we want to fathom the greatest treasures hinted at in the t'ai chi diagram.

Everyone deserves the chance to develop to their fullest potential. We have a profound responsibility to provide opportunities to help our colleagues, friends, family and coworkers to gain a Three-in-One outlook on their situation through expanding the container of their awareness. We're all, in varying degrees, proficient in the field of the Three. What is missing is a familiarity with the One. There are two fullnesses to life, one inner and silent (the One), and the other outer and active (the Three). Unless we have both, we're living a very limited version of what is possible. A profound scientific discovery during the 1970s was that, in fact, only a very small proportion of any population is needed to function with greater measures of awareness in order to change the trends of time towards greater positivity for everyone. There is a wealth of scientific and statistical evidence to show that we are all deeply connected on the plane of consciousness. The benefits of growth of awareness don't accrue to the individual alone, but influence the surroundings at the most fundamental and the most global levels also.

Once we have located the source of consciousness, the abode of Tao, in our own awareness, then we can use a ***samyama*** practice to stir it up at the level of the Gap. Action initiated at this level enjoys the support of all the laws of Nature. It is the level of complete inclusiveness. Nothing is left out or forgotten, everything, everywhere and every time is spontaneously considered—so there are no mistakes. Spontaneous right action is the basis of a happy and fulfilling life. The sequence is to first capture the One in our awareness and then to integrate it into our everyday activity, the arena of the Three (through the practice of t'ai chi, for example). 1-in-3. It only works in that order.

Coherent brain functioning spreads orderliness through the environment as a field effect in consciousness. This is a well-researched phenomenon. When just a small number of individuals are consciously operating from the level of the Gap, the very innocent byproduct of their success is a spontaneously happy and peaceful world. This effect is the sublime expression of the martial arts. Averting the danger that has not yet come.

LOOKING THROUGH THE EYES OF NATURE

As a result of cultural conditioning, we all have our own beliefs about what happens at the end of this life. Some believe that they are going to Heaven. Others think that after a brief rest it's back on the reincarnation treadmill until they've earned their place in Heaven. Still others are of the opinion that all this clinging to the idea of a separate and enduring individual identity is a bit of a farfetched case of self-importance. No matter their beliefs, most people are somewhat daunted by the thought of dropping their bodies.

In the end, all views are simply belief systems. No one *knows* because, by definition, one's nervous system can not go through the actual experience and remain there. It could be argued that the high level of similarity of reports of "near death experiences" points to nothing more than an artifact of the normal progression of the nervous system shutting down. In the early days of the first runs of "Quick Draw McGraw", when you turned your TV off, a bright glow appeared and lingered in the middle of the screen—just an artifact of the equipment before the advent of spot suppression circuitry.

With the usual pragmatic vision, the martial artist asks: "How do you prepare a warrior to face, with calmness, *sente* and fearlessness, the prospect of imminent death on the battlefield?" One answer is to provide a small taste of "death" by using extended cerebral hypoxia (oxygen starvation in the brain) as a result of a carotid choke out. For a while, the participant is kept under this deeply unconscious condition in order to experience "the other side." I have been led through the procedure under the guidance of a skilled master (it is very dangerous to do this without an expert facilitator). Consumed in blissful transcendence, I was completely unaware of what was happening with my body on the physical plane. It was like a very deep but lively meditation. However, when dealing with transcendence we're dealing in the field of wu chi, ***samhita***, the field of the One, the simplest form of awareness and the ground state of consciousness. In other words, in a realm beyond space and time—making it impossible to definitively correlate the subjective event with the entire time that my body was disabled. Like the well-publicized near-death experiences, my brief journey was profound and the fear of death greatly ameliorated, but this is still no proof that anything exists for us other than the present.

In the final analysis, all we have is all anyone ever had since the beginning of time—the Now. By practice and training, aligning ourselves with the t'ai chi diagram, by being established in conscious awareness of the One in the midst of the Three, we can attain the Tao here in this moment. We claim our birthright in the deathless Pure Intelligence and Existence from which our life began, which sustains us, and into which we return at the end—all without ever leaving it. By operating through the "eyes" of the diagram, by acting from within the Gap at the juncture of relative and absolute, we gain the status of the divine. We evolve to be the conscious authors of our manifest destiny, stewards of the world, making full use of the talents given to us. And thus we are truly…

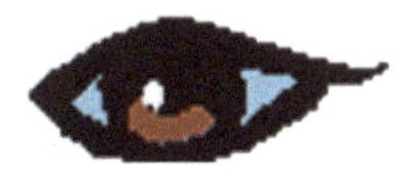

Looking Through the Eyes of Nature.

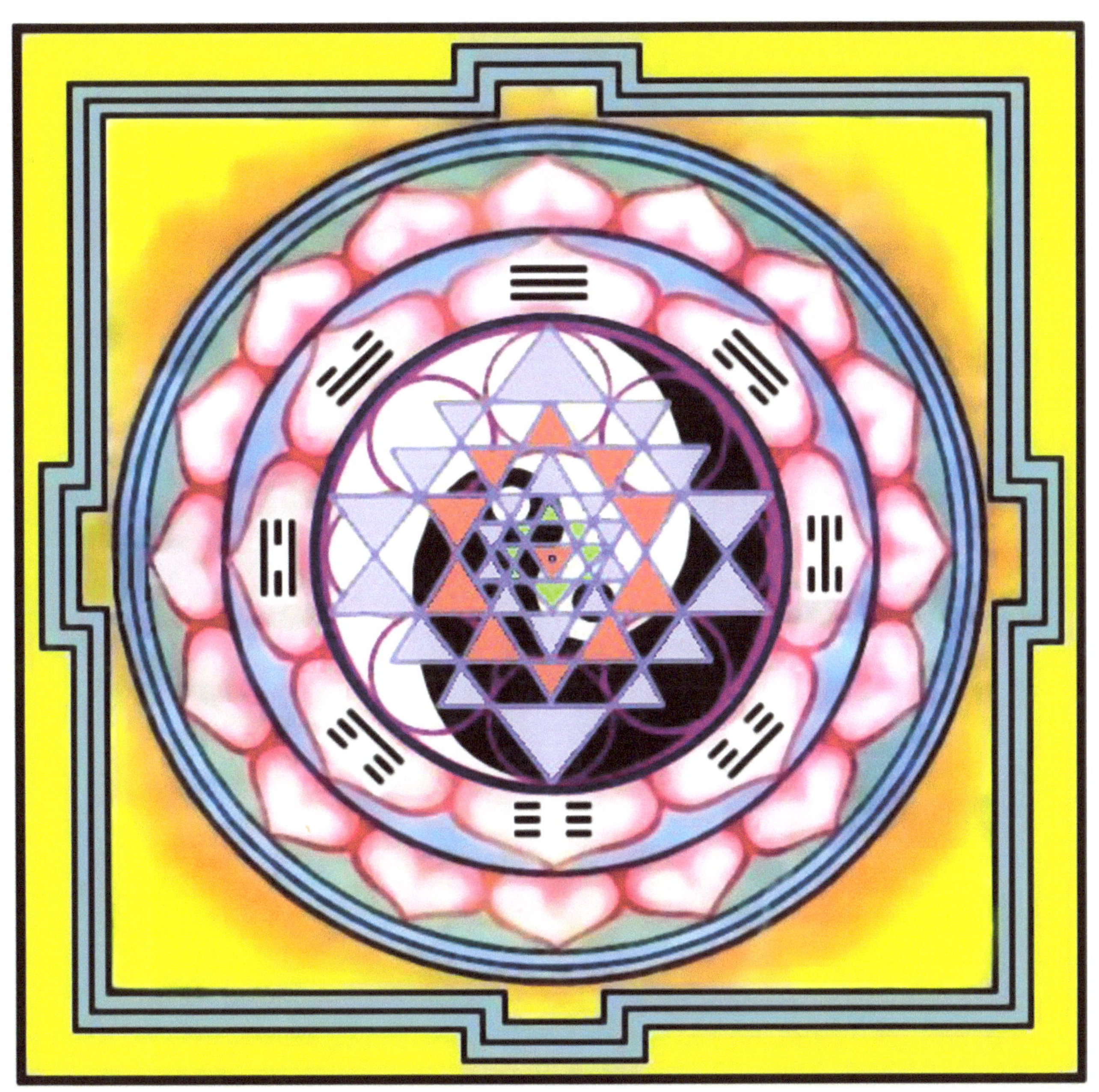

ABOUT THE AUTHOR

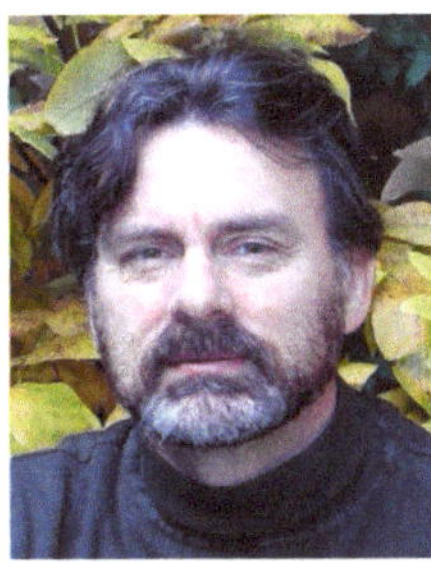

In this, his first book, Max Wright talks about the 3-in-1 nature of reality from his life-long experiences in the martial arts and development of consciousness.

The recurring theme of three has featured predominantly in his personal life also, from growing up in England, to coming of age in South Africa, to a mid-life immigration to the US.

The three parallel and enduring streams of his adult years have comprised a deep involvement in both the practice and teaching of meditation, a passionate love of the eastern martial arts, and a successful professional career in computer information processing consulting.

The three members of his American family are his wife and two children. Max lives in the Ozarks of NW Arkansas.

www.ingramcontent.com/pod-product-compliance
Lightning Source LLC
LaVergne TN
LVHW070133110826
845147LV00002B/242
9781421899640